FIRST PLACE BIBLE

LIVING
in GRACE

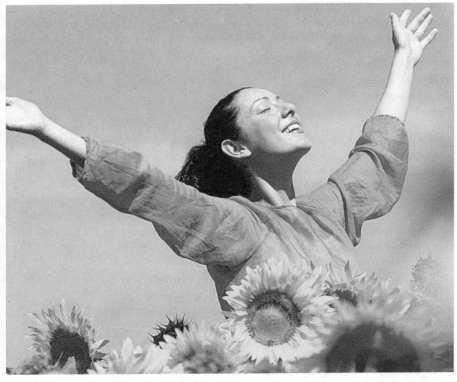

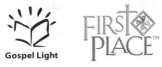

Gospel Light

FIRST PLACE™

Gospel Light is an evangelical Christian publisher dedicated to serving the local church. We believe God's vision for Gospel Light is to provide church leaders with biblical, user-friendly materials that will help them evangelize, disciple and minister to children, youth and families.

It is our prayer that this Gospel Light resource will help you discover biblical truth for your own life and help you minister to others. May God richly bless you.

For a free catalog of resources from Gospel Light, please contact your Christian supplier or contact us at 1-800-4-GOSPEL or www.gospellight.com.

PUBLISHING STAFF

William T. Greig, Chairman • **Bill Greig III,** Publisher • **Dr. Elmer L. Towns,** Senior Consulting Publisher • **Natalie Clark,** Product Line Manager • **Pam Weston,** Managing Editor **Patti Pennington Virtue,** Associate Editor • **Hilary Young,** Editorial Assistant **Jessie Minassian,** Editorial Assistant • **Bayard Taylor, M.Div.,** Senior Editor, Biblical and Theological Issues • **Rosanne Moreland,** Cover and Internal Designer • **Denise Munton,** Contributing Writer

Songs: Written and produced by Keith Mohr, Jamie Harvill, Joe and Theresa Mazza and Ed Kerr. Vocals: Jason Barton, Candace Hargett, Missi Hale, Theresa Mazza, Michelle Gold, Mia Kim, Ritchie Crook and Jamie Harvill. Voice-overs: Mia Kim and Eric Luedtke. Production supervised by Keith Mohr, Broken Records Productions **http://www.brokenrecords.com**

CAUTION

The information contained in this book is intended to be solely informational and educational. It is assumed that the First Place participant will consult a medical or health professional before beginning this or any other weight-loss or physical fitness program.

CONTENTS

FOREWORD

My introduction to Bible study came when I joined First Place in March of 1981. I had been in church since I was a small child, but the extent of my study of the Bible had been reading my Sunday School quarterly on Saturday night. On Sunday morning, I would listen to my Sunday School teacher as she taught God's Word to me. During the worship service, I would listen to our pastor as he taught God's Word to me. Digging out the truths of the Bible for myself had frankly never entered my mind.

Perhaps you are right where I was back in 1981. If so, you are in for a blessing you never dreamed possible. As you start studying the truths of the Bible for yourself, you will see God begin to open your understanding of His Word. Bible study is one of the nine commitments of the First Place program. The First Place Bible studies are designed to be done on a daily basis. Each day's study will take approximately 15 to 20 minutes to complete, but you will be discovering the deep truths of God's Word as you work through each week's study.

There are many in-depth Bible studies on the market. The First Place Bible studies are not designed for the purpose of in-depth study. They are designed to be used in conjunction with the other eight commitments of the program to bring balance into our lives. Our desire is for each member to begin having a personal quiet time with God each day. This time alone with God should include a time of prayer, Bible reading and Bible study. Having a quiet time is a daily discipline that will bring the rich rewards of balance, something we all need.

A part of each week's study is the Bible memory verse for the week. You will find a CD at the back of this Bible study that contains all 10 of the memory verses for the study set to music. The CD has an upbeat tempo suitable for use when exercising. The songs help you to memorize the verses easily and retain them for future reference. If you memorize Scripture as you study, God will use His Word to transform your life.

Almost every First Place member I have talked with about the program says, "The weight loss is wonderful, but the most important thing I have received from my association with First Place is learning to study God's Word."

God bless you as you begin this exciting journey toward a balanced life. God will richly bless your efforts to give Him first place in your life. Remember Matthew 6:33: "But seek first his kingdom and his righteousness, and all these things will be given to you as well."

Carole Lewis
First Place National Director

INTRODUCTION

The First Place Bible studies were developed to be used in conjunction with the First Place weight-loss program. However, the studies could also be used by anyone who desires to learn more about God's Word and His will, with the added bonus of learning more about living a healthy lifestyle.

A Balanced Life

First Place is a Christ-centered health program, emphasizing balance in the physical, mental, emotional and spiritual areas of life. The First Place program is meant to be a daily process. As we learn to keep Christ first in our lives, we will find that He is the One who satisfies our hunger and our every need.

God's Word contains guidelines for maintaining our physical well-being, equipping us mentally to make right choices, providing emotional stability to handle everyday circumstances as well as crisis situations and growing spiritually as we deepen our relationship with Him.

The Nine Commitments

The First Place program has nine commitments that will help you draw closer to the Lord and aid you in establishing a solid, consistent and healthy Christian life. Each commitment is a necessary and important part of the goal of First Place to help you become healthier and stronger in all areas of your life—living the abundant life He has planned for each of us. To help you achieve growth in all four areas, First Place asks you to keep these nine commitments:

1. Attendance
2. Encouragement
3. Prayer
4. Bible reading
5. Scripture memory verse
6. Bible study
7. Live-It plan
8. Commitment Record
9. Exercise

The Components

There are six distinct components to this Bible study to aid you in bringing balance to your life. These components include the 10-week Bible study, a Wellness Worksheet, 2 weeks of menu plans, the leader's discussion guide, 13 Commitment Records and the Scripture Memory Music CD.

The Bible Study

Each week of each 10-week Bible study is divided into five daily assignments with Days 6 and 7 set aside for reflections on the week's lesson. The following guidelines will help make your study more enjoyable and profitable:

- Set aside 15 to 20 minutes each day to complete the daily assignment. It's best not to attempt to complete a week's worth of Bible study in one day.
- Pray before each day's study and ask God to give you understanding and a teachable heart.
- Keep in mind that the ultimate goal of Bible study is not only for knowledge but also for application and a changed life.
- First Place suggests using the *New International Version* of the Bible to complete the studies.
- Don't feel anxious if you can't seem to find the *correct* answer. Many times the Word will speak differently to different people, depending upon where they are in their walk with God and the season of life they are experiencing.
- Be prepared to discuss with your fellow First Place members what you learned that week through your study.

Wellness Worksheet

This study's Wellness Worksheet is interactive and will help you learn to accurately determine exchanges in each of the seven food-exchange groups.

Menu Plans

The two-week menu plans were developed especially for First Place by Chef Scott Wilson. Each menu is meant to simplify meal planning and include food exchanges. These meals are based on the MasterCook software that uses a database of over 6,000 food items and was prepared using United States Department of Agriculture (USDA) publications and information from food manufacturers.

Leader's Discussion Guide

This discussion guide is provided to help the First Place leader guide a group through this Bible study. It provides information for the leader to prepare for each weekly group meeting.

Personal Weight Record

The Personal Weight Record is for the member to use to keep a record of weight loss. After the weigh-in at each week's meeting, the member will record any loss or gain on the chart.

Commitment Records

Thirteen Commitment Records (CRs) are provided in the back of this Bible study. For your convenience these have been printed on perforated paper so that you can easily remove them from the book and carry them with you through each week as you keep your First Place commitments. Directions for filling out the CRs precede those pages.

Scripture Memory Music CD

Since Scripture memory music is such a vital part of the First Place program, the Scripture Memory Music CD for this study is included in the back inside cover. The verses for this study are set to music that can be listened to as you work, play or travel. The CD can be an effective tool as you exercise since the first verse is set to music with a warm-up tempo, the next eight verses are set to workout tempo, and the music of the last verse can be used for a cooldown.

THE GOD OF ALL GRACE

God wants you to live a fulfilled life (see John 10:10). It is His desire that you experience His love and grace every day and that you understand how the freedom you can experience through a relationship with Him will affect every area of your life: spiritual, mental, emotional and physical. If you believe and receive the truth, you have unlimited access to the supernatural healing power of God's grace *and* everything you need to defeat the enemy.

In this week's study, you will discover how your heart and mind can be transformed through the work of the Holy Spirit when you acknowledge, confess and surrender your life to the Lord *daily*. Jesus Christ empowers us to live victoriously.

DAY 1: *The Freedom of God*

Through the sacrifice of His Son, Jesus, God has given you freedom. Let's explore what that freedom means.

➤ According to Galatians 5:1, from what has Jesus freed you?

The word translated as "freedom" in this verse means that your freedom has been purchased.

➤ What was the purchase price for your freedom?

➤ Note the command to "stand firm, then, and do not let yourselves be burdened again by a yoke of slavery." What kinds of things keep us burdened under the yoke of slavery to sin?

➤ In what area(s) of your life are you enslaved and burdened? Be specific. Ask the Holy Spirit to reveal what's holding you captive, thus hindering your intimacy with the Lord.

But how can we get out from under those things that enslave us? Let's look at God's Word. "And I will walk at liberty and at ease, for I have sought and inquired for [and desperately required] Your precepts" (Psalm 119:45, AMP).

➤ According to Psalm 119:45, what is the prerequisite for walking in freedom, or liberty?

Through desperately seeking God's Word, we become empowered to walk away from old habits and the slavery of sin and to run *into* God's freedom, liberty and grace.

When you begin to walk in freedom, your life will never be the same. You will be transformed into the person God has called you to be, and your transformation will be apparent to others in your life. Your cares in this world will diminish as you begin to look forward to spending time with your heavenly Father. As you learn more about

Jesus Christ, you will love Him like never before—and you will be free to love not only yourself but also others with His love.

Father God, I confess my sinful and unbelieving heart that turns me away from You, the living God. Help me to encourage those around me daily so that none of us may be hardened by sin's deceitfulness.

Thank You, Jesus, that when I hold firmly to my trust in You, I can daily rest in Your freedom and peace [see Hebrews 3:12-14].

DAY 2: *The Word of God*

Everything you think and do is a direct result of what you believe. Your measure of belief determines your actions, and your actions determine how you live your life. If you want to change how you respond to life and relationships, you must first determine what it is that you believe.

According to Hebrews 4:12, what is the Word of God?

What does the Word penetrate?

What does it judge?

God's Word is alive! It is quick and powerful, penetrating your heart and revealing the truth. God's Word brings health and healing to your mind and body, discerning your motives, thoughts and attitudes.

➤ Take a moment to think about your reactions to and belief in the Word of God. Do you believe every word of the Bible is alive and active? Please explain.

Isaiah 55:10-12 is a beautiful illustration of what happens to God's Word when it is sent forth! When you pray the Word, you are praying God's perfect will. You don't have to wonder if you are asking Him for something that He won't do.

If you have any doubt about what the Bible is saying to you, stop and pray, confessing your unbelief and asking for the Holy Spirit's wisdom and understanding. The enemy's weapon of unbelief will no doubt continue to challenge you each step of the way, but you are not without weapons on the road to freedom in Christ.

➤ According to 2 Timothy 4:16-18, who stood beside Paul and gave him strength when everyone else had deserted him?

What is the promise found in verse 18?

➤ Use the following scale to rate your belief in the promise of the Lord to rescue you:

1	2	3	4	5
Weak		So-So		Strong

≫ As you read Philippians 4:13 and 2 Timothy 4:17, what one word ties these two verses together?

In these passages, the word translated "strength" indicates a power that comes from within. When you are faced with difficult circumstances and you can't seem to find any way out, God's Word will go forth and empower you to forge ahead. When you are at your lowest or weakest point, the Holy Spirit will empower you. Your circumstances may not change, but your outlook and attitude will. Isaiah 26:3 and James 1:6-8 give us additional encouragement as we seek His Word for strength.

Dear Father, You have given Your Word to help me know You. I don't want to be tossed like a wave at sea—let Your words penetrate my inmost being, that they may dispel any doubt I have that You are willing and fully able to sustain me with Your strength [see James 1:6].

DAY 3: *The Transforming Power of God*

One of the keys to being transformed and obtaining freedom is found in Mark 11. Before you go forward today, stop and ask the Lord to open your heart so that you can know the truth. Then ask Him for the strength to act upon that truth in the name of Jesus Christ.

≫ In Mark 11:24-25, what is the connection between answered prayer and forgiveness?

Why do you think that forgiving others is so closely tied to answered prayer?

➤ Ask the Holy Spirit to bring to your mind anyone whom you need to forgive. This could be someone who has wronged you intentionally or someone whose actions hurt you but perhaps he or she doesn't even know it. Write down that person's first name or initials and what it is that you need to forgive him or her for.

Not only do we need to forgive others, but we also need to seek forgiveness from those we have hurt or wronged.

➤ Ask God to reveal anyone from whom you need to seek forgiveness. Write down that person's first name or initials and what it is that you need forgiveness for. Plan on when and how you will ask this person's forgiveness.

Remember, this is key to your freedom and transformation. If you're not sure you can give or seek forgiveness, ask God to soften your heart and to give you the strength and power to walk in obedience. When you trust and believe God's Word, obedience is a natural response.

➤ As you read Philippians 3:12-14, what is the Holy Spirit revealing to you? Do you want to press forward, leaving behind the hurts from the past?

Choose today to lay down all your fears, doubts and your unbelief. Pick up the baton—the Word of God—and run with all your might toward your goal. Don't look back! When you attempt to overcome sin and obstacles with only your own power and reasoning, you will struggle and fail.

Read Philippians 3:13 again. You must deliberately stretch yourself as you move toward your goals. In your pursuit, He will require obedience on your part. If you sense an unwillingness to obey, pray again for God to empower you. Confess that there are areas in which you are weak, areas that make you uncomfortable or afraid and areas in which you need a lot of strength.

> O God, You are the master of transformation. Change me through the power of Your Word, for it is life to my whole body [see Proverbs 4:22].
>
> Father, as I learn to submit to Your transforming power, teach me to guard my heart, which is the wellspring of life [see Proverbs 4:23].

DAY 4: *The Armor of God*

As you draw nearer to the Lord, the devil will fight back. He will do everything in his power to defeat you and to keep you from experiencing God's grace and freedom. He would love to steal your joy and liberty by causing you to drag along the chains of legalism, insecurity or disobedience. Fortunately, you have already been given the weapons you need to arm yourself against the devil's lies and deceitful schemes. As Paul described in Ephesians 6:10-18, when you put on the full armor of God, you are prepared to stand your ground and not run in fear.

➣ What two pieces of armor are we instructed to put on first (v. 14)?

Everything you speak and do needs to be said and done in truth— and truth only comes from God's Word. At the same time, when you are surrendered to God and clothed in righteousness, your heart is protected. The enemy has no way in.

➣ What piece of armor should be put on after truth and righteousness (v. 15)?

We live in a world filled with anything but peace; however, we are empowered by the Holy Spirit to take the gospel of grace and peace into the world.

≫ What is the purpose of the next piece of armor, the shield of faith (v. 16)?

The "flaming arrows" can include fear, doubt, unbelief, unforgiveness or any lie or temptation that comes your way.

≫ What are the final two pieces in the full armor of God (vv. 17-18)?

The helmet of salvation protects your mind, and the sword of the Spirit defends you against the lies with which the devil tries to deceive you. Your mind is where the battle begins. Ask the Holy Spirit to help you recognize the lies that the devil tries to put in your mind. You must deliberately reject deceitful thoughts, recognizing them as lies; then tear down the lies by replacing them with truth from God's Word. Reprogram your mind by learning God's Word. Pray continually, using the truth that is the sword of the Spirit.

≫ According to James 4:7, what two things must we do when the enemy comes against us and what will happen as a result?

John 8:44 tells us that the devil "was a murderer from the beginning, not holding to the truth, for there is no truth in him. When he lies, he speaks his native language, for he is a liar and the father of lies."

≫ According to 1 Peter 5:8-10, what might you endure in order that you may be restored and made strong, firm and steadfast?

You have to choose to resist and stand firm against the schemes of the devil. If you try to ignore him, you will be deceived.

➤ What does Jesus say about Himself in John 10:10?

Jesus Christ came so that we might have life to the full, or—as the *King James Version* and the *New King James Version* translate it—"abundantly." God is not just interested in helping you survive. He wants to give you a quality of life that only He can give—an abundant life full of peace and joy.

Father, I thank You that though I live in the world, I do not wage war as the world does. The weapons You have given me have divine power to demolish strongholds and every pretension that sets itself up against the knowledge of You. Father, help me take every thought captive and obedient to You [see 2 Corinthians 10:4-5].

DAY 5: *The Peace of God*

➤ According to 2 Corinthians 12:9, what did the Lord promise Paul concerning his weaknesses and infirmities?

You may be familiar with this verse, but when you experience it personally, it is so real and powerful. When you feel defeated or when circumstances seem overwhelming, you may cry out, "Oh, God, I'm so tired! I don't understand this, I want to quit. I want to give up—I can't handle this anymore!" Then with a deep breath, you continue, "But I trust You, Lord." At that moment, remember His promise: "My grace is sufficient for you, for my power is made perfect in weakness" (2 Corinthians 12:9). God is in control and is at work even when you don't see it.

➤ Philippians 4:6-7 describes how you can obtain the peace of God. What is your part in the process?

What does His peace do?

This indescribable, supernatural peace is beyond all comprehension. When others look at you, knowing the circumstances you are facing, they are either dumbfounded or are greatly encouraged because they see the power of God in your life. Instead of whining and grumbling about your circumstances, you can wear a garment of peace, grace and joy, which is seen and felt by others.

➤ In John 14:27, what did Jesus promise?

➤ What are some areas that you are troubled or fearful about and, therefore, not entrusting to God?

Claim Jesus' promise of peace for those things that trouble you.

 O God, thank You that since I have been justified through faith, I have peace with You through my Lord, Jesus Christ. It is through Jesus that I have gained access to the grace in which I now stand [see Romans 5:1].

As I present my requests before You, O God, guard my heart and mind with Your peace—a peace that the world cannot comprehend [see John 14:27; Philippians 4:6-7].

DAY 6: *Reflections*

In your pursuit of freedom, you will struggle with bouts of unbelief. You will be tempted to turn around and cower under your former beliefs that enslave you to fear, pride, self-centeredness, self-condemnation, unforgiveness, defeat, etc. But God, in His faithfulness, will continue to pursue you, to reveal truth, as you request wisdom and understanding. As you search the heart of God and pray His Word, you will begin to see and experience His power in your life. Suddenly, the things you previously tried to control and the things you have worried yourself over will become insignificant. The burden of self-gratifying and self-striving will lift.

If you are struggling with a particular area in your life that is causing you to feel enslaved, you need to face that circumstance, that problem, that fear and rely on God's strength to overcome. It is only through prayer and God's Word that you will gain the strength to break the bonds of slavery.

One way to learn to pray more effectively is to pray using God's Word. Praying through Scripture is the process of taking a verse and praying it back to God in your own words. Beth Moore's book *Praying God's Word* explains the process.[1]

The process isn't complicated: You take a particular verse and pray that verse to the Lord, personalizing the words. The following are examples of praying Scripture:

> You, Lord my God, are merciful and forgiving, even though I have rebelled against You. Help me also to be merciful and forgiving to others [see Daniel 9:9].[2]
>
> Lord God, give me more grace so that I may increasingly extend it to others [see James 4:6].[3]
>
> Blessed am I because my transgressions are forgiven. Blessed am I because my sins are covered. May my deep gratitude be evident in the way I relate to others, O Lord [see Psalm 32:1].[4]

DAY 7: *Reflections*

As you know, freedom does not come without opposition. There will be days when you feel insecure and defeated. Fear, doubt, unbelief and temptation will continue to try to gain a foothold. When you feel these things, know that you are literally in the midst of a battle for your freedom. Allow the Holy Spirit to rise up within you and say no to the enemy. Don't give up—and don't ignore these attacks. Stand your ground and take action, using the full armor of God to defeat the enemy (see Ephesians 6:10-18).

On the road to weight loss and healthy living there will be ups and downs, but the difference when you are walking with the Lord is that the valleys aren't as deep as when you walked alone. Now, by the grace of God, when you stumble or feel weary and wounded, you don't have to give up. Instead, you can simply run back into the arms of Jesus. One of the ways to do that is to open His Word and seek His comfort and direction.

"Now the Lord is the Spirit, and where the Spirit of the Lord is, there is freedom" (2 Corinthians 3:17). God has so much to give us in His Word. Earnestly pray as you study the Word that you would hear, receive and act on what the Holy Spirit reveals to you. Pray that the Holy Spirit will fill you, empower you and transform you into His likeness. Ask your heavenly Father to surround you with the presence and the power of His peace. You have absolute access to this freedom, regardless of who you are or what you have done. Receive it in the name of Jesus!

I love You, O Lord, my strength! You are my rock, my fortress and my deliverer; You, my God, are my rock, in whom I take refuge. You are my shield and the horn of my salvation, my stronghold! I call to You, O Lord, who is worthy of praise, and I am saved from my enemies [see Psalm 18:1-3].[5]

Some trust in chariots and some in horses, but I trust in the name of You, the Lord my God. My enemy will be brought to his knees and ultimately fall, but I will rise up and stand firm [see Psalm 20:7-8].[6]

Father God, I thank You that because I am in Christ, Satan, the prince of this world, has no hold on me [see John 14:30].[7]

Notes

1. Beth Moore, *Praying God's Word* (Nashville, TN: Broadman and Holman, 2000).
2. Ibid., p. 229.
3. Ibid., p. 232.
4. Ibid., p. 228.
5. Ibid., p. 314.
6. Ibid., p. 316.
7. Ibid., p. 326.

GROUP PRAYER REQUESTS   TODAY'S DATE:_____

NAME	REQUEST	RESULTS

OUR SIGNIFICANCE TO GOD

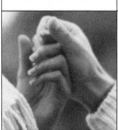

MEMORY VERSE

*For you created my inmost being; you knit me
together in my mother's womb. I praise you because
I am fearfully and wonderfully made; your works
are wonderful, I know that full well.*

Psalm 139:13-14

In this week's study you will discover how significant you are to the God
of all grace. Do you know just how deeply loved, accepted and cherished
you are by your heavenly Father? As you earnestly continue forward in the
freedom race, you will take with you some very special and personal truths
from God's Word, and you will be empowered to encourage others in
their race.

DAY 1: *God's Love*

John 3:16 is probably the most recognized and memorized verse in the
entire Bible. This powerful verse reveals God's love and purpose for the
world. Not only was God referring to mankind as a whole, but He was
also referring to each one of His children specifically. You are one of His
children.

➤ According to Romans 4:25, what was the purpose of Jesus' death and
resurrection?

Read Romans 5:6-8. Have you ever thought that your love for someone was so deep that you would die to protect that person? Most of us
have. Imagine, then, a love so powerful that you would willingly take the
place on death row for someone who was guilty beyond doubt—someone

who wasn't even sorry for his or her sins! Hard to imagine, isn't it? Yet, that is exactly what Christ did.

➣ Take a moment to think about a time when you really felt God demonstrate His love for you. Briefly explain the experience and how you felt knowing you were loved so much.

According to Psalm 139:1-18, nothing about you is a surprise to God. You were made by Him! Nothing you go through is beyond God's reach; His light can shine into any darkness. He is with you in everything you do, from the tedious details to the life-changing events—every moment of your life is important to Him.

➣ How does God's incredible love for you affect your desire to follow the First Place commitments?

Remember Romans 5:8? Do you understand the depths of God's love for you? He loves you no matter what. As you go through your day and struggle to make healthy and wise choices, remember how much Christ loves you and what He has already done for you.

Dear Father God, my heart overflows with gratitude because of Your incredible love for me. Thank You for demonstrating Your grace by choosing to love me and calling me to Yourself even though I was dead in sin [see Romans 5:8].

Loving Lord, give me the power to understand just how wide and long and high and deep Christ's love is for me—a love that surpasses knowledge! [see Ephesians 3:17-19].

DAY 2: *God's Direction*

Psalm 139:3 (*NLT*) says, "You chart the path ahead of me." Did you know that God has a plan for your life? He knows what will happen to you today, tomorrow and in your future—and the encouraging part about that is that He loves you more than anyone else does!

≫ According to Matthew 10:29-30, how well does God know you?

Psalm 139:15-16 says that not only did God form you, but He is also constantly at work in your life.

≫ Describe a time when you have experienced God at work in your life, directing or protecting you in some specific way.

≫ According to Proverbs 3:5-6, what will happen when we acknowledge the Lord in *everything* we do?

We are all guilty of relying on our own understanding. We assume that we know what's best for us—which path will be the straightest. But our own knowledge and experiences are limited. Why wouldn't we commit our plans to the One who sees and knows everything? He is the only One who can make our path straight!

≫ What does John 15:9-11 tell us about how Jesus loves us?

How do you remain in His love?

>> What will your belief, obedience and trust in God ultimately bring?

Describe a time in your life when you experienced this supernatural joy as a result of obedience, even if obeying wasn't the easiest choice.

>> What is one area of your First Place commitments in which you need to be more obedient?

No matter where life's journey takes you, Christ's joy completely satisfies and supplies your emotional and spiritual needs. Stop focusing on your circumstances and start looking up to Jesus. He will empower you to stand, endure and remain steadfast and obedient on the path that He is guiding you to follow.

Father God, You are familiar with all my ways. You know me intimately! Help me to trust that You also know what is best for me, that You will only set me on paths that will draw me closer to You [see Psalm 139:3].

Loving Shepherd, You promise to guide me along the best pathway for my life. Help me trust that You will advise me and watch over me [see Psalm 32:8].

Thank You, Lord God, that I can trust You completely. I never have to rely on my own understanding, for You will make my paths straight [see Proverbs 3:5-6].

DAY 3: *God's Rest*

Psalm 139:3 (*NLT*) states, "You . . . tell me where to stop and rest. Every moment you know where I am." God is even concerned that you take time to rest. He knows where you are, what you are dealing with and what you need right now. He has even commanded us to rest (see Exodus 20:8-11)!

➵ According to Matthew 11:28-30, what does Jesus offer to do for you?

➵ What must you do to receive the rest that you are offered?

Resting in Jesus does not necessarily mean that you will be removed from circumstances, trials, activities or responsibilities. It means that as you submit to the power and authority of Jesus and commit your situation to Him, you are connected to Him and He bears the weight of your burden. He shares in your suffering. Resting in Him empowers you to remain steadfast no matter the circumstances.

➵ Is there something in your life that is so deeply burdening you that you've become weary and in need of rest? Write it down here and then commit the situation to the Lord.

It can be hard to give our troubles over to God for Him to handle. Often we give a situation over to Him only to take it back. Ask God to show you how to give this burden to Jesus to carry for you, and each time you try to take it back, ask Him to help you to trust Him to take care of it.

➵ According to verse 29, why is Jesus willing to take on your burdens?

≫ What happens to your burdens when you give them to Jesus (v. 30)?

You may feel that learning the Live-It plan and keeping the other eight commitments are burdensome, but knowing that Jesus is there to help you will be an encouragement. Ask Him to help you keep your commitments and your load will be lightened.

Thank You, God, for never tiring of taking my burdens. Give me the strength to exchange my heavy load for Your light one. Teach me what it means to be gentle and humble, like Your Son, Jesus Christ [see Matthew 11:28-30].

Father, Your compassion never fails; it is new every morning! Great is Your faithfulness! You, Father God, are good to those whose hope is in You, to the one who seeks You. Father, help me place my hope in You and seek You alone [see Lamentations 3:22-25].

DAY 4: God's Provision

Yesterday, you learned about giving your heavy burdens to Jesus and taking up His yoke. Today you are going to look into the heart of *Jehovah Jirah*, your God and your provider.

≫ In Genesis 22:1-18, Abraham faced the ultimate test of obedience to the Lord when he was told to sacrifice Isaac. Can you think of a time when obeying the Lord was painful? Explain how you were ultimately blessed by your obedience.

When Abraham told his servants that he and Isaac would be back (v. 5), he was confessing his belief in the promise that he had been given in Genesis 21:12: "It is through Isaac that your offspring will be reckoned." Although he was willing to obey God's command to sacrifice his son,

Abraham knew that somehow God would make good on His promise.

➤ Have you been given a promise from the Lord for which you are still waiting? Have you tucked it in the back of your mind or forgotten it because you think it won't happen? Write down that promise and claim it again.

➤ Have you ever had to place one of your dreams or desires on the altar as a sacrifice in obedience to the Lord? Please explain.

In today's society, there is a mind-set that tells us we are entitled to have all that the world has to offer and to have it *now*. As the world continues to place more importance on material possessions, professional success and wealth, God is steadfast in His command that we trust in Him, seeking His will for our lives. The world is in direct opposition to the life that God has for you.

➤ Read Matthew 6:24-25. In what situations are you most likely to be ruled by your physical desires?

➤ According to Matthew 6:33, what must you do to be free from worldly concerns? How does that apply to your commitments in First Place?

Freedom of any kind does not come without a struggle, and this is especially true of breaking free from worry over your physical needs. You do not have to face this battle alone, however.

➤ What are the promises found in 1 Corinthians 10:13?

➤ Take a moment to pray and ask the Holy Spirit to reveal areas of worry in your life that might be hindering your intimacy with Jesus. Write down those areas here and pray Philippians 4:6, asking the Lord to forgive you for being anxious about worldly concerns.

God empowers you to stand up against the lies of the world, lies that tell you that the things the world has to offer are more exciting and satisfying than what God has for you. When you yield and submit your will to Him, seeking His face in every situation, He will give you more than you could ask for or imagine. When you give your whole heart to Jesus, His desires become your desires. As a result, you can rest assured that all of your needs will be met by Him. God knows what you need and when you need it. His timing is perfect. Trust Him!

Search me, Lord, and know my heart; test me and know my anxious thoughts. See if there is any offensive way in me, and lead me in Your ways [see Psalm 139:23-24].

I praise You, Jehovah Jirah, because You know all my needs and will meet each one according to Your glorious riches in Christ Jesus [see Philippians 4:19].

Thank You, Father, that I can never be lost from Your Spirit. Empower me now by Your Holy Spirit to relinquish control of my life, to surrender it to You and allow You to meet my every need. God, I trust You!

DAY 5: *God's Protection*

When you love something, you'll do everything you can to protect it from harm. David knew that the Lord loved him, and he also knew that he needed divine protection from his many enemies—even from his own volatile emotions. Throughout the Psalms, we see examples of David crying out for the protection that only God could provide. His prayers reveal different ways that God protects His children.

➤ Read Psalm 25:21. How can integrity and uprightness protect you?

➤ In Psalm 40:11, David asked the Lord to protect him with His love and truth. Describe a time when you have been protected by the truth of God's Word.

In Psalm 69:29 the Hebrew word for salvation, *yeshuw`ah*, can also be translated "deliverance" or "victory."[1] Perhaps it's time we pray as David did, asking God to protect us by delivering us from—and giving us victory over—our strongholds! But you might ask, What is a stronghold?

Beth Moore tells us that a stronghold may be an addiction, an unforgiving spirit toward a person who has hurt us or despair over loss; and it demands so much of our emotional and mental energy that our abundant life is strangled. You, too, can break down the spiritual strongholds in your life as you pray through the Scriptures.[2]

➤ What are the promises in Psalm 121?

➤ According to Proverbs 3:5-6, what is the prerequisite for straight paths?

When you trust in the Lord and lean on Him, you can be confident that He will lead you in the right direction.

➤ According to Proverbs 2:1-11, whom does God guard and protect?

What is our part in God's protection?

As you pursue your relationship with the Lord, ask Him daily for His wisdom, knowledge, understanding, insight and discernment. Because of His great love for you, He promises protection, direction, provision and rest, if you seek Him and submit to Him wholeheartedly.

Lord of the night watches, You never tire of watching over me! Your eye is ever on me, and You will not let my foot slip [see Psalm 121:3-4].

Father, help me preserve sound judgment and discernment. Then I will go on my way in safety; my foot will not stumble. When I lie down, I will not be afraid, and my sleep will be sweet [see Proverbs 3:19-24].

DAY 6: Reflections

When you read the promises found in Psalm 139:17-18, it can be hard to accept that God is always with you. You may even feel at times that you are the exception to this truth—that God isn't interested in what's going on in your life. Or you might have moments when you doubt God's love and acceptance of you because past sins come to mind. Nothing could be further from the truth.

When you have thoughts of doubt and unbelief, ask the Holy Spirit to help you identify the enemy's lies and hold on to the truth. At that moment, you must consciously take up your sword of truth and begin confessing that truth with your mouth. Through Scripture memorization, you can arm yourself with the truth that will always defeat the lies of the devil.

When thoughts of doubt or memories of past sins cause you to want to give up following Jesus, stop and confess Romans 8:1: "Therefore, there is now no condemnation for those who are in Christ Jesus." Praise the Lord for His wonderful plans for your life. The enemy will flee, your mind will clear, your heart will lift, and you will walk forward in freedom!

Lord God, help me to trust in Your unfailing love. Cause my heart to rejoice in Your salvation. Help me to sing to You, Lord, for You have been good to me! [see Psalm 13:5-6].[3]

O God, please set my heart at rest in Your presence when my heart wants to condemn me. For You, God, are greater than my heart, and You know everything [see 1 John 3:19-20].[4]

Father God, how great is the love You have lavished on me, that I should be called a child of God! And that is what I am! [see 1 John 3:1].[5]

DAY 7: *Reflections*

Remember Matthew 11:28-30?

> Come to me, all you who are weary and burdened, and I will give you rest. Take my yoke upon you and learn from me, for I am gentle and humble in heart, and you will find rest for your souls. For my yoke is easy and my burden is light.

As you keep your eyes fixed on Jesus, you'll begin to reflect His characteristics of gentleness and humility. When you become gentle and humble, you are not only reflecting His grace, but your whole attitude, perspective and outlook regarding your circumstances also begin to change.

Your heavenly Father has given you victory through Jesus and His awesome love for you. He sent His Holy Spirit to comfort you and reveal the truth in times of struggle. You mean so much to Him. He has given you everything you need to live on this earth while He prepares a place for you in heaven. His grace and love are sufficient for you to accomplish all He asks of you (see 2 Corinthians 12:9). Don't stop, don't give up, and don't look back! Keep your eyes on Jesus Christ and your ears focused on God's Word.

Lord, many are the woes of the wicked, but Your unfailing love surrounds the one who trusts in You. You are so trustworthy, God. Please help me to place my complete trust in You [see Psalm 32:10].[6]

You, the Lord my God, are with me, You are mighty to save. You will take great delight in me, You will quiet me with Your love, You will rejoice over me with singing! [see Zephaniah 3:17].[7]

You, O Lord, love me with an everlasting love; You have drawn me with loving-kindness. You will build me up again and I will be rebuilt. I will take up my tambourine and go out to dance with the joyful! [see Jeremiah 31:3-4].[8]

Notes

1. "The KJV Old Testament Hebrew Lexicon," *Crosswalk.com*. http://bible.crosswalk.com/Lexicons/Hebrew/heb.cgi?number=03444&version=kjv (accessed June 25, 2003).
2. Beth Moore, *Praying God's Word* (Nashville, TN: Broadman and Holman, 2000), p. 3.
3. Ibid., p. 92.
4. Ibid., p. 95.
5. Ibid., p. 96.
6. Ibid., p. 105.
7. Ibid., p. 107.
8. Ibid.

GROUP PRAYER REQUESTS   TODAY'S DATE:_____

NAME	REQUEST	RESULTS

WHAT IS GRACE?

How would you describe God's grace? It is a term that Christians often use, but if you asked several Christians what grace means, you would probably get as many definitions as the number of people you ask! One common definition is "unmerited favor." *But what does that mean?*

This week's study will provide you with a better understanding of God's grace and your need for it. Allow the Word to wash over you and change your life as you take in these truths!

DAY 1: *A Priceless Treasure*

What is something that is priceless to you—something that you would not part with for any price? Is it a treasured heirloom? Would you name your family or friends as your priceless treasures? God has paid for our sin with His most priceless treasure—Jesus.

➤ How is Jesus described in Hebrews 1:3?

What did Jesus accomplish before He took His place at the right hand of God in heaven?

Before Christ took His rightful place in heaven, He placed Himself on the altar as an offering for our sin so that we might have a relationship with the Father.

➤ Continue reading Hebrews 1. Does this change your view of who Jesus is? Please explain.

Romans 1:20-23 reminds us that humankind has known from the beginning that God is our creator, but we have consistently turned our backs on Him, worshiping things instead of worshiping the One who created us.

Read Romans 1:28-32. What a sad picture of humankind's sinful nature! You may be thinking to yourself, *I'm not that bad! I'm not wicked, and I certainly haven't* murdered *anyone!* The truth of the matter is that it is our inherently sinful nature that makes us unworthy of a relationship with God. God doesn't compare your sin with the sins of others because sin *is* sin to God.

➤ How does it make you feel to know that even the *worst* sins are forgivable? Do you think this is fair? Please explain.

➤ When you realize that you can receive God's forgiveness regardless of your past sins, how does that affect you?

➤ Some might think that we can do anything we want and just ask forgiveness afterward, and our gracious God will continue to forgive. What does Romans 6:1-2 say about this attitude?

How might this wrong thinking affect your choice to persevere in your First Place commitments?

Do you make excuses for your wrong choices? *Well, just this once I'll eat the rest of the cookies; then tomorrow I'll exercise longer.* Or *I'm just so busy today; I'll skip my Bible study time this morning and catch up tomorrow.* The problem is that when we consciously make a bad choice, it is easier to give in next time; and then we begin to feel defeated and give up easily.

Although each sin brings its own consequences, sinning is what keeps you from a relationship with God, but—praise Jesus!—He forgives the murderer just as He forgives the gossip. It doesn't matter that we try to be good; we will never be good enough to enter heaven until we allow Jesus Christ to cleanse us of our sins, fully accepting Him into our lives. "Here I am! I stand at the door and knock" (Revelation 3:20). Let Him in!

Dear God, help me comprehend and embrace how You loved me first by sending Your one and only Son into the world in order that I would live through Him [see 1 John 4:9-10].

Jesus, You are the radiance of God's glory and the exact representation of His being, sustaining all things by Your powerful Word; You now sit at the right hand of the Majesty— our Father—in heaven. I bow my heart before You in awe, for You have redeemed me! [see Hebrews 1:3].

Thank You, Father, that You have offered me the precious treasure of Your grace in Jesus' sacrificial death on the cross for *my* sin.

DAY 2: *A Free Gift*

God's grace-filled love is a gift to us. We have done nothing to deserve it; in fact, if we had to earn God's love, it would be impossible. We are completely dependent upon His mercy and His grace.

What does Romans 3:20-24 say about how have we been justified?

It can be hard to accept the truth that God loves you just as you are and that you don't have to do anything to prove yourself worthy of His grace. He offers it as a free gift.

According to Ephesians 2:8-9, why can't we earn God's grace?

What are some ways in which you have tried to earn God's love, attempting to ensure that you remain in His grace?

What does Ephesians 2:10 say about the relationship between God's grace and the good works we do?

How easy it can be to reverse that order! We think that we must somehow earn God's favor by doing certain things before we are saved; instead we need to continually remind ourselves that His grace is a gift.

What is the promise found in 2 Corinthians 5:17?

In the first two weeks of this study, we talked about identifying and resisting the lies of the enemy. The enemy wants you to believe that the promise of 2 Corinthians 5:17 is a lie. He wants you hang on to your past and never forget your mistakes or sins. If you allow the enemy to convince you that your feelings are true and that the Word is a lie, you have given him a foothold and he will imprison you with his deceit.

↠ According to 2 Corinthians 5:14-15, how are we to live?

What is at least one specific way that you can live your life for Christ this week?

If you are struggling with the lack of desire and motivation to follow Christ, tell Him exactly how you feel. It is important to remember that although God already knows everything about you, including your thoughts and feelings, it is only through your confession of those thoughts and feelings that He can begin to work to change your heart toward Him.

If you have previously accepted Jesus into your heart but have been walking in complacency or disobedience, remember that God wants to help you find your way back to Him. Before you can succeed in any area of your life, including meeting your goals in the First Place program, you have to make sure your heart is right with God. Sheer determination and willpower fail every time. Start asking God today, and then every day, for a renewed desire and excitement to follow after and spend time with Him.

Lord God, make the reality of Your abundant grace vivid in my heart today. I know there is nothing I could ever do to earn Your favor, and yet You lavish me with many blessings. All I can do is humbly thank You.

Help me, Jesus, to show my gratitude by fleeing from sin and pursuing righteousness, godliness, faith, love, endurance and gentleness [see 1 Timothy 6:11].

DAY 3: *An Expressive Faith*

Let's take a look again at Abraham, a man considered righteous by God (see Genesis 15:6; Romans 4:22). Long after Abraham and his wife, Sarah, were beyond their childbearing years, God promised to give them a son (see Genesis 15:4). Abraham immediately believed that God would do as He said. Even though the fulfillment of this promise took many years, Abraham continued to have hope and believed that God would not forget His promise. Finally, when Abraham was over 100 years old, he became a father. Years later, when Abraham was told by God to offer his son Isaac as a sacrifice, Abraham set out to do what he was told—all the while remembering God's promise that through Isaac, the descendants of Abraham would become a great nation (see Genesis 17:19) and believing that God would allow Isaac to live.

➽ Considering Romans 4:13-15, why is it more important to have faith than to simply obey the rules?

➽ What is the value of a promise to someone who has no faith? Why?

Having faith in God means believing that He will do everything He has said He would. Over and over again God has proven faithful to His promises; He has never failed. He has given us more than enough evidence that He is the creator of all things and that He only desires what is best for us. All we have to do is believe it, receive it and act on it!

➽ Use the following scale to rate your measure of faith.

1	2	3	4	5
Weak		So-So		Strong

➣ Read Romans 10:9-10. Why do you think that it is important not only to have faith in your heart but also to confess aloud what you believe?

➣ How does James 2:18-23 relate to acting on your faith?

How does acting on your faith relate to keeping the Nine Commitments in First Place?

Hebrews 11:6 states, "without faith it is impossible to please God." Do you want to please Him? What do you need to trust Him for? The verse continues: "Anyone who comes to him must believe that he exists and that he rewards those who earnestly seek him." Will you earnestly seek the Lord today and every day this week?

Father, help me not waiver in unbelief regarding Your promises. Strengthen my faith to give glory to You [see Romans 4:20].

O God, I desperately need to meet with You every day. Give me the desire, excitement and motivation I need to seek You and to read Your Word daily. God—Redeemer, Savior, Friend, Companion—empower me to walk by faith!

DAY 4: A Transforming Power

Although it is impossible for any human being to live a sinless life—no matter how dedicated he or she is to serving God—this knowledge does not give us free rein to do as we please and take the grace God extends for granted.

≫ According to Romans 6:1-7, when you accept Christ as your Savior, why should you not continue to live a sinful life?

How is living a sinful life different from sinning in moments of weakness?

A Christian who chooses to continue living a sinful life is willfully and consistently sinning despite what he or she knows about Christ. That person is making a conscious choice to walk through life with God at arm's length, allowing Satan to maintain a foothold.

≫ According to Romans 6:14, why is sin no longer the master of your life when you walk with Christ?

≫ What is the result of believing in the Lord Jesus Christ and having been set free from sin (see Romans 6:20-23)?

The fact is that until you get to heaven, you will struggle with sin. But you are not without resources to resist sin. The Holy Spirit empowers you to withstand the temptations of the enemy (see Ephesians 6:13). God gave you free will to choose between sin and righteousness. At those times when you fall, run back into Jesus' arms, confess your sin, turn around (the actual meaning of "repent") and proceed forward once again. Jesus loves you so much that He is thrilled when you jump back into His arms. When those who live under guilt and condemnation fall, they stay down, feeling unworthy and unloved, which results in losing the race.

≫ According to Romans 12:1-2, what must you do to *not* conform to the patterns of this world?

When something is transformed, it undergoes a complete change. When something is renewed, it is made new again. Not only does a relationship with God completely change you, but God will also make you new again! What a great promise!

≫ What are you able to do when you have been transformed and renewed (v. 2)?

When your life is in sync with God's will and you earnestly seek Him every day, you will avoid the pitfalls that giving into temptation can cause. Jesus Himself experienced temptation (see Matthew 4:1-11).

≫ According to Matthew 4:1-11, what did Jesus use against Satan when tempted in the wilderness?

Instead of giving in, Jesus relied upon the Word of God and eventually the devil left in defeat. Remember James 4:7: "Submit yourselves, then, to God. Resist the devil, and he will flee from you."

If there is an area of addiction or a stronghold in your life, counseling may be necessary. However, if your counselor doesn't use the ministry and counsel in God's Word, you will be wasting your time. There is no counselor, teacher, minister, method or technique apart from the Word of God that can set you free.

 Gracious Lord, I know that the life I now live is through Your Son, Jesus Christ. I will not set aside Your grace by thinking that I can earn my righteousness by the good things I do [see Galatians 2:20-21].

O Father, You called me to be free. Keep me from using my freedom to indulge my sinful nature, but help me serve others in love [see Galatians 5:13].

I am Christ's ambassador because I have been reconciled to You, O God. Help me live my life in such a way that others will be drawn to You as well [see 2 Corinthians 5:20].

DAY 5: *Freedom from Guilt*

If you have accepted Christ and received forgiveness yet continue to live with feelings of guilt and condemnation, the enemy still has a foothold in your life. Though he has lost rights to your soul and he knows you will live forever in the kingdom of God someday, Satan will do everything in his power to keep you from the peace, hope and joy that you are entitled to here on Earth.

➤ Compare Romans 8:1-4 and 2 Corinthians 7:8-11. What is the difference between condemnation and godly sorrow?

To what does godly sorrow lead? To what does worldly sorrow lead?

➤ Why are Christians not condemned?

➤ Most people who need to lose weight continually deal with feelings of guilt or shame regarding the bad choices that have led them to their present unhealthy condition. Are you dealing with feelings of guilt or shame about anything in your past? Confess these feelings to the Lord.

Allow today to be a pivotal point. Rather than growing weak and weary under Satan's lies and accusations, you can stand your ground, confess the truth and render him powerless. Drive a stake into the ground. Today, you acknowledge that you have been forgiven and you walk out of the open prison door to freedom, never to return.

Help me, O God, to throw off everything that hinders me—including guilt and shame—so that I may run with perseverance the race marked out for me. Keep my eyes fixed on You, Jesus! [see Hebrews 12:1-3].

Lord, cause my godly sorrow to lead me to repentance. May it produce an earnestness and longing for You so that even my past mistakes work for Your ultimate glory [see 2 Corinthians 7:10-11].

Thank You, Father, for forgiving my transgressions and covering my sins. I am blessed because my sin will never count against me! I choose to walk out of the opened door of my prison cell and live as a free child of Yours—never to be enslaved again! [see Romans 4:7-8].

DAY 6: *Reflections*

In this week's study, you have discovered the importance and wonder of God's grace. Jesus loves you and gives His grace freely. Humbling your heart every day is key to living in that grace. Earnestly pray for a desire to spend time every day with the Lord because of His awesome and unconditional love for you, not because it makes you a *good* Christian. Pray the Word with all your heart—especially when you don't feel like it!

➤ What does Hebrews 4:12 say about God's Word?

God's Word is alive and powerful. If you are struggling with fully believing the Word of God, confess this truth to the Lord and continue to ask Him to cause His Word to penetrate your heart and wash away your unbelief.

As you pray for wisdom, knowledge, understanding, insight and discernment, use the weapons you have been given to walk in freedom. In doing so, you will begin to experience less time in the pit of guilt and shame and more time in the peace and grace of God.

Lord, Your inspired Word declares that the knowledge of Your truth leads to godliness [see Titus 1:1].[1]

Father God, help me to give You great joy by walking in the truth, just as You commanded us [see 2 John 4].[2]

Father God, continue to teach me. Help me to recognize what is in accordance with the truth that is in Jesus [see Ephesians 4:21].[3]

DAY 7: *Reflections*

Ephesians 2:8-9 says, "For it is by grace you have been saved, through faith—and this not from yourselves, it is the gift of God—not by works, so that no one can boast." Are you serving God, trying to do all the right things, yet lacking the peace and intimacy you want with Him? It can be easy to fall into the mind-set of legalism and not even realize it. Before you know it, you are setting standards and rules for yourself that only bind you rather than free you.

Consider that the foundation you have built this week has been set in stone. It has been established deep in the ground. Humbly pray that you will receive and believe the awesome grace that Jesus so lovingly purchased for you by His blood. Even though it was a high price, God would have it no other way. All you have to do is receive His Grace and believe His Word. As a result of faith, you have received the promised Holy Spirit, and have been made a coheir with Jesus. You can now walk upright, filled with the presence of God.

My Lord, Your Word is right and true; You are faithful in all You do. You love righteousness and justice. I thank You that the earth is full of Your unfailing love! [see Psalm 33:4-5].[4]

Ah, Sovereign Lord, You have made the heavens and the earth by Your great power and outstretched arm. Nothing is too hard for You! [see Jeremiah 32:17].[5]

For me, there is but one God, the Father, from whom all things came and for whom I live; and there is but one Lord, Jesus Christ, through whom all things came and through whom we live [see 1 Corinthians 8:6].[6]

Notes

1. Beth Moore, *Praying God's Word* (Nashville, TN: Broadman and Holman, 2000), p. 82.
2. Ibid., p. 83.
3. Ibid., p. 81.
4. Ibid., p. 32.
5. Ibid., p. 26.
6. Ibid.

Group Prayer Requests   Today's Date:_____

Name	Request	Results

HINDRANCES TO GRACE

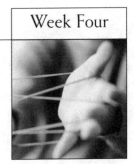

MEMORY VERSE

See to it, brothers, that none of you has a
sinful, unbelieving heart that turns away from
the living God. But encourage one another daily,
as long as it is called Today, so that none of
you may be hardened by sin's deceitfulness.
Hebrews 3:12-13

So far in this study we have discussed who God is, who we are in Christ and what grace is. Unfortunately, understanding these things isn't enough. You can still sabotage yourself from partaking in God's grace by allowing sin to hinder you. In this week's study we are going to look at the hindrances to experiencing God's grace so that you can be on your guard to not forfeit the blessings He wants to lavish on you.

DAY 1: *Unbelief*

Unbelief is the weapon that Satan uses to hinder us from grasping the reality of God's Word. When we allow the enemy to steal our belief in God's promises, we will be rendered powerless and live in sin and defeat.

One of the ways to combat unbelief is to exercise our commitment to memorize Scripture. When we hide God's Word in our heart, the Holy Spirit recalls the Word to our mind in times of need, especially in times of spiritual battle as we resist temptations to sin.

➤ According to Hebrews 3:12-15, what turns our hearts away from the living God?

➤ Describe when you have experienced a time that you were "hardened by sin's deceitfulness." What was the result of that experience?

Abraham's faith in God was amazing. If you are fully persuaded of the truth that God is who He says He is and has power to do what He has promised, your life will reflect it in the same manner as Abraham's life did. Not only will you experience God's power, but you will also live righteously.

➤ Read Hebrews 3:8-11. Why was the disobedience of Israel so disturbing to God?

What does verse 14 say we must do in order to share in Christ?

In Deuteronomy 10:21, Moses reminded the Israelites that they had seen God perform "great and awesome wonders" with their own eyes and not to forget God or take Him for granted.

➤ Briefly describe when you first accepted Christ. How sure were you of what you believed at that moment?

In what way have you lost your confidence in Christ (see Hebrews 3:14)?

Your steadfast belief will determine whether you live righteously or defeated. Are you willing to "hold firmly till the end" (Hebrews 3:14) to the faith you had when you first believed, or are you going to allow your life to be controlled by unbelief? Will you walk obediently or in disobedience?

When you overcome unbelief, your life will display God's grace and power and will be credited to you as righteousness.

O God, I confess the unbelief in my heart. Help me, God, to stand firm and believe every word that I hear through Your Word [see Isaiah 7:9].

Precious Jesus, though I have not seen You, I love You. And even though I do not see You now, I am filled with inexpressible joy because I believe in You [see 1 Peter 1:8].

Help me, Lord, to be good soil in which the seed of Your Word will be firmly rooted. Help me to retain it and nurture it, keeping it free from the thorns of unbelief [see Luke 8:12-15].

DAY 2: *Fear*

There are two kinds of fear mentioned in the Bible. The first is fear *of* God and the second is fear that stems from *not trusting* God. Fear of God causes us to obey His commands "so that we might prosper" (Deuteronomy 6:24-25). This is an awe and a respect for God that recognizes His power, authority and His holiness.

Fear that comes from not trusting the Lord keeps us from experiencing His grace. The Bible tells us that this fear, or timidity, is not from God (see 2 Timothy 1:7). As subtle as it can be, fear has the potential to render you powerless. Fortunately, you have been given the means to overcome this destructive fear.

➵ Take a closer look at 2 Timothy 1:7. What spirit does God give you?

When Jesus leads you to do something, whether you believe you can do it or not, He gives you the ability to do it if you obey by faith. When you begin thinking *I can't do that*, you can be sure that the enemy is trying to instill the fear that paralyzes you and keeps you from trusting God.

≫ Describe a time in your life when fear paralyzed you. How were you able to overcome your fear?

When you are sensing God's direction but begin to feel fearful, you have a choice to make. Read the story of Elijah in 1 Kings 17:1-16.

≫ When Elijah met the widow at the town gate, what did he ask her for (vv. 10-11)?

What was the widow's reply to Elijah's request (v. 12)?

When Elijah told the widow to use what she had to make enough bread to feed three people, she must have thought he was out of his mind! After all, she barely had enough to feed herself and her son one last time. Nevertheless, because God had commanded the woman to feed Elijah (v. 9), she did as she was asked. She had faith in Elijah's promise that God would provide more (vv. 13-14).

≫ What might have happened if the woman had given in to fear and not fed Elijah with the last of her family's food?

➤ Have you ever faced a situation in which you needed to do something that defied all logic and required you to take a leap of faith? What was the result?

➤ Right now, are you facing something that you fear? Write your fear here. Examine it and confess it to the Lord, asking for His power to overcome it.

An accurate acrostic for fear is False Evidence Appearing Real. Sometimes, that which we fear most doesn't even exist. The widow in the story you just read had nothing to fear because God had promised to provide for her. Any fears she may have entertained were just lies from the enemy, fabricated to torment her into disobeying the Lord.

If you allow fear to control your life, it will be impossible to experience and administer God's grace. It hinders your intimacy with Jesus, and as a result, you live in defeat and are blinded to the truth.

 O God, I confess I have allowed fear to hinder my obedience to You. [Name the areas causing fear.] I praise You, God, that You have not given me a spirit of fear but a spirit of power, love and self-discipline [see 2 Timothy 1:7].

Father, empower me by Your Holy Spirit to step out in faith—just like the widowed woman—believing You will accomplish through me that which You have called me to do.

DAY 3: *Critical Spirit*

Judging others can be easy to do—and it's definitely easier than assessing our own faults! As a matter of fact, let's try an illustration. Take your hand and point your finger outward. Now turn your wrist and point that same finger toward yourself. It's a little more uncomfortable to do, isn't it? It is the same way with criticism, and a critical spirit can keep us from experiencing God's grace.

≫ According to Matthew 7:1-5, why should we not judge others?

≫ What does James 1:26 warn us about our tongue?

Most of us can remember times that we have been the recipient of someone else's unreined tongue. We can probably remember times that we have allowed our tongues to run free. It is hurtful to relationships when we do not keep our tongues under the control of the Holy Spirit.

≫ What does James 4:11-12 say about judging others?

What are we doing when we are judgmental toward others?

Have you ever been involved in gossip? Of course, you have— you're human. Gossip can be very tempting, even for Christians. For example, let's say a friend is having marital problems and comes to you in confidence for advice and prayer. When that friend doesn't show up to small group the next week, you become concerned. During prayer time, you decide to tell the group what's going on so that everyone can pray for your friend. You might have the right intentions, but it's still gossip. Gossip is a form of judging others.

>> What do you think about a person who gossips about others? Would you tell that person details about your life? Why or why not?

>> What steps could you take to avoid the sin of gossip and still ask for prayer for your friend in the previous example? Be specific.

Remember that you are in a battle. You have to deliberately choose to sow righteousness. It is natural for us, in our flesh, to criticize and gossip; but remember that although your flesh reacts naturally, God has empowered you to respond supernaturally.

If you are dealing with a critical spirit, begin today to acknowledge it and confess it before the Lord. Ask the Holy Spirit to convict your mind every time you are about to criticize or gossip. Ask Him for the strength to speak praises with your mouth instead of slander. If you slip and fall, jump up and brush yourself off; then run back into the arms of Jesus. Don't allow condemnation to come in and convince you that you'll never change. Cling to the truth that you have God's supernatural power to do what is right.

O Holy God, I bow my heart in submission to You. I confess my critical spirit and the gossip I've been involved in toward [state person's name].

Thank You, Father, for Your cleansing and forgiveness. Help me to slander no one, but instead be peaceable and considerate, and to show true humility toward all [see Titus 3:2].

Help me pray Your Word for people that I've slandered. I want to see them through Your eyes and love them with Your love. In the name of Jesus, amen!

DAY 4: *Unforgiveness*

Forgiving someone who has hurt you can be one of the hardest things to do. The truth is that without God you simply can't do it. Be assured that if you *don't* forgive, you will be trapped in a harbor through which healing will not flow, and you will be hindered from experiencing the fullness of God's grace.

➤ According to Matthew 6:14-15, why are we commanded to forgive others?

➤ In Luke 23:34, what did Jesus pray just before He died on the cross?

Why did Jesus ask the Father to forgive the people who crucified him?

Jesus, the Son of God, had been ridiculed, beaten, bruised and nailed to a cross; but having experienced more pain than you could ever imagine, He asked His Father to forgive those who crucified Him. He had every right to hate them for what they had done, but He didn't. In reality, He was dying for them too!

➤ How does Matthew 5:43-44 relate to forgiveness?

Why do you suppose Jesus related forgiving others to the forgiveness we receive from the Father?

When you are unforgiving of others, they are not being punished—you are. You are the one holding on to the pain, allowing it to harden your heart. When you live with a hardened heart, every relationship you have is affected, including your relationship with God.

➤ According to Ephesians 4:26-27, what happens when you hang on to anger and unforgiveness?

Is there someone toward whom you harbor unforgiveness? Are you willing to let go of the unforgiveness you hold toward this person? Seek godly counsel and begin to allow the Holy Spirit to minister to your heart. Healing doesn't come overnight; it is a process. Someone once said that forgiving someone is not dependent on feelings, but it is a conscious choice we must make.

As you continually choose to forgive—completely surrendering to Christ—you will experience His grace and peace like never before. Stop a moment and sit quietly before the Lord. Ask Him to speak to your heart and to help you learn to forgive.

 My Father God, help me to see and understand the power of Your forgiveness. I confess my unforgiveness toward [state person's name] and need Your help to forgive.

As Your dearly loved and chosen one, clothe me with compassion, kindness, humility, gentleness and patience. Help me bear with others and forgive whatever grievances I have against them. For I choose to forgive as You, Lord, have forgiven me [see Colossians 3:12-13].

DAY 5: *Envy*

If you have children, you know from experience that the envious nature is revealed at a very young age. Even as toddlers, children whine, cry and reach for any toy that another child has. For some reason that baby doll in little Mary's arms looks much more appealing than the one Cindy is grasping in her own pudgy fingers! Although adults don't show their envy as openly as children do (most of the time!), we never completely outgrow our childish ways.

Harboring any envious thought or feeling can hinder us from experiencing God's grace. When our eyes are focused on the things we don't have, we overlook all the magnificent blessings God has given us—blessings tailor-made for our individual needs. God knows that the human heart is naturally envious, but He also wants us to experience the peace and joy that comes with true contentment. That's why He warns against envy, or coveting, in the Ten Commandments (see Deuteronomy 5:21).

➣ How might envy prevent you from keeping the commandment in John 15:17?

In our materialistic society, it is easy to assume that when we envy someone, it's for material possessions. But we can be envious of other things too: another person's lifestyle, relationships or even spiritual gifts. What about envying another person's body type? Have you ever felt a tinge of jealousy that your friend can eat anything she wants and never gain a pound, yet your hips widen when you even smell sweets? This type of envy may seem harmless at first, but its effects are detrimental in the long run.

➣ What do you think Solomon meant when he wrote in Proverbs 14:30 that envy "rots the bones"?

When you compare who you are or what you have to others, there are only two possible outcomes: Either you will be overcome with envy because they have what you think you want, or you will become puffed up with pride. Neither of these is a Christlike response.

You've no doubt heard the popular phrase "the grass is always greener on the other side." But the darker hue you perceive is either an illusion or the result of a lot of hard work. Remember that nothing is exactly the way it appears at first glance, including people's seemingly easier lives. You have no way to know what another person is dealing with emotionally, mentally, physically or spiritually. If you envy a friend for her perfect body, realize that while she may appear to have it all together, appearances can be deceiving—she could be looking at you, wishing she had something that you have. Or perhaps it only seems that she can eat what she wants when in fact she carefully balances out her daily food choices and exercises a lot to maintain her weight and health.

➤ According to 1 Timothy 6:6-8, what is considered great gain?

It's impossible to be content when our eyes are focused on ourselves and our selfish desires. But when we focus on Christ, this world and everything in it fades away. We brought nothing into this world, and we can take nothing out—not even our earthly bodies!

As children of the most high God, we have more reason than anyone to be content. We know that we are wonderfully and fearfully made and that the maker of the universe knit us together to be just who we are (see Psalm 139:13-14). Don't let envy rob you of the grace God wants to lavish on you as His child.

Father, I confess my sin of envy—of comparing myself to others. But in my heart of hearts, I trust You to meet all my needs. Help me die to my selfish ways, that I may trust You more fully.

Great Provider, give me neither poverty nor riches, but only my daily bread. Otherwise, I may have too much and disown You and say, "Who is the Lord?" Or I may become poor and steal, and so dishonor Your name, my God [see Proverbs 30:8-9].

Teach me the secret of being content in every situation, knowing that You, my God, will meet all my needs according to Your glorious riches in Christ Jesus [see Philippians 4:12-13,19].

DAY 6: *Reflections*

In this week's study, we focused on five hindrances to experiencing God's grace. These crucial areas keep you not only from experiencing grace but also from extending it to others.

There are four steps you can take to combat every hindrance: (1) Put on the armor of God; (2) confess having yielded to that hindrance—when the spirit of fear or any other temptation comes upon you and you yield to it, it becomes sin; (3) take the shield of faith and resist the spirit of fear or that temptation in the name of Jesus; and (4) take the sword of the Spirit and confess the truth out loud (see Ephesians 6:13-17). Seek God's wisdom every day in dealing with those things that threaten to hinder you from experiencing His grace. Ask the Holy Spirit for help so that you will recognize every hindrance and for His power to say no to those hindrances so that you will walk in obedience.

Right now, ask the Holy Spirit to reveal the things in your life that keep you from an intimate walk with Jesus. Give those things over to the Lord. Remember 1 Corinthians 10:13: "No temptation has seized you except what is common to man. And God is faithful; he will not let you be tempted beyond what you can bear. But when you are tempted, he will also provide a way out so that you can stand up under it." Stand on that promise as you pray for help.

Christ Jesus, You said, "The work of God is this: to believe in the one he has sent" [John 6:29]. That is what You want from me more than anything in the world.[1]

Father, as You did for the jailer who received salvation through the witness of Paul and Silas, fill me with joy when I choose to believe [see Acts 16:34].[2]

DAY 7: *Reflections*

This week's Scripture memory verse reminds us of the importance of encouraging each other daily. God has placed us in a family of believers for a reason. Although through the Holy Spirit you have all the weapons you need to wage war against Satan's lies, the battle is much easier when we fight it together.

There are two reasons why we need to encourage one another daily. The first is to keep one another accountable. It's much easier to detect when a brother or sister in Christ is giving in to a subtle lie than to detect it in ourselves. Likewise, a brother or sister may detect signs of a hardening heart in us long before we ever realize it.

The second reason is that through encouragement we can cheer one another along during the tough times. Just as a football team rallies when the fans cheer them on, we need others to shout encouragement to carry us through the difficult times.

Always remember: You have been forgiven and can walk in the freedom of God's grace. You also have the encouragement of others who are right there fighting the battle beside you. No longer should unbelief, fear, unforgiveness, a critical spirit and envy hinder God's grace in your life. Though everybody's circumstances may differ, the precepts and principles of God's Word are the same for everyone. As you daily confess your heart attitude and the sins that hinder God's grace in your life, you will walk in freedom. As you pray the living and active Word of God, you will live renewed and transformed, walking in the light of victory and God's glory. You are free, beloved!

Christ Jesus, Your Word tells me to be on my guard, to stand firm in the faith, to be a person of courage and to be strong [see 1 Corinthians 16:13].[3]

Lord God, please place someone in my path who will travel with me for my progress and joy in the faith [see Philippians 1:25].[4]

Lord, please help me to flee the evil desires of youth and pursue righteousness, faith, love and peace, along with those who call on the Lord out of a pure heart [see 2 Timothy 2:22]. You want me to pursue faith, not just sit back and wait until it develops.[5]

Notes
1. Beth Moore, *Praying God's Word* (Nashville, TN: Broadman and Holman, 2000), p. 42.
2. Ibid., p. 43.
3. Ibid., p. 49.
4. Ibid., p. 50.
5. Ibid., p. 52.

GROUP PRAYER REQUESTS   TODAY'S DATE:_____

NAME	REQUEST	RESULTS

THE PROCESS OF GRACE

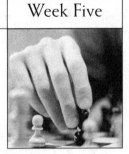

MEMORY VERSE

*This righteousness from God comes through faith
in Jesus Christ to all who believe. There is no difference,
for all have sinned and fall short of the glory of God,
and are justified freely by his grace through the
redemption that came by Christ Jesus.*

Romans 3:22-24

Although God views us as righteous because of Christ's work on the cross, we are a long way from being perfect in our daily lives. That's why God extends another aspect of His grace: our sanctification. Sanctification is another gracious gift from God, but it is a lifelong process. Christ's work on the cross cleansed us on the inside, but we must still undergo the process of becoming holy and pure on the outside. In this week's study we are going to explore a few of the elements of the sanctifying process of grace.

DAY 1: *Acceptance*

When we choose Christ as our Savior and decide to follow Him whole-heartedly, God accepts us as we are, and He no longer views us as fallen sinners. Instead, He sees us just as He sees His holy and perfect Son, Jesus Christ. This week's memory verse, Romans 3:22-24, makes it clear that we can do *nothing* to earn that righteousness—it only comes by God's grace and we only need to accept His gift. In His infinite grace, God imparts to us the righteousness of His Son! There's nothing we can ever do to earn it!

➤ What did Jesus ask His disciples to do in Matthew 4:18-22 and 9:9?

The Greek word translated "follow" in verse 19 is *deute* which means "come hither," "come here" or "come now."[1] There is no prerequisite to your coming. Jesus says, "Come now! I don't care what you've done or where you've been. Just come as you are, and I will make you my disciple." Simon Peter, Andrew, James and John weren't model saints when Christ called them; they were your average, rough-around-the-edges fishermen! But they came, nonetheless—faults and all.

As a believer, do you hesitate to completely surrender your life to Christ because you feel there are areas in your life you must get together first? Or as an unbeliever, are you trying to prepare yourself, trying to change some things in your life or otherwise attempting to make yourself ready because it is hard to believe that God accepts you and calls you from where you are at this moment?

>> Pray, asking the Holy Spirit to reveal those things that need to be left behind. Write down what the Holy Spirit is bringing to your mind. Be honest and specific.

The *King James Version* of Matthew 4:20 reads, "And they straightway left their nets, and followed him." The Greek word *eutheos* translated "straightway" means "immediately."[2] This is how we need to respond to His call. The moment He reveals Himself, the moment the Holy Spirit reveals Truth is when we need to respond, whether it is coming to know Jesus or simply obeying whatever He is directing us to do.

>> When you are compelled to do something, how often do you stop to contemplate whether or not you really heard from God? Check all with which you can identify.

 ☐ I discuss the situation with friends and mentors, getting their advice to try to figure out what I should do.

 ☐ I tend to be passive-aggressive, pretending I did not hear Him or sometimes shrugging it off, trying to convince myself it is not a big deal.

 ☐ I sometimes wrestle with God because I am not ready, I don't feel like it or I just refuse to do it.

 ☐ I pray, search the Word, wait and listen for the Holy Spirit's guidance and direction on what to do next.

➤ When we are disobedient to the Lord's direction, we needlessly take on a heavy load. Is there something in your life that you sense God has been directing you to do, but you have been making excuses? Write down those things that are coming to your mind. You can trust that the Holy Spirit is speaking to you right now.

➤ Why do we struggle with the concept that God loves us as we are and that we do not need to win His love?

Remember, the enemy doesn't want you to come to the Father just as you are, because he knows if he can keep you in denial or fear, he's got you and your lack of freedom right where he wants it: in his clutches. Fight for your freedom! Ask God to help you obey Him and know clearly what He is directing you to do. Then do it!

O Father, my heart of hearts longs to walk obediently, but my sinful flesh is so strong! Father, I confess my disobedience in these areas: [state them]. Empower me now by Your Holy Spirit to do the things that I now know I am supposed to do.

Your Word declares that I can do all things through Christ who gives me strength. O God, I cry out for Your strength and I choose to walk in obedience [see Philippians 4:13].

Jesus said that when I receive Your commands and obey them, I am one who loves You. And greater still, You will love me and show Yourself to me [see John 14:21].

Jesus accepted you just the way you were when you came to Him. Then He began the process of cleansing and changing you.

To repent means to change your direction and abandon your personal agenda. This obviously applies to new believers when they come to know Jesus. At the same time, repentance also applies to those who already know and follow Him. Throughout this study, you have been instructed to confess your sin over and over again. In doing so, you are acknowledging your sin, changing your direction and abandoning your agenda, not because you need to be saved again, but because you live in a sin-infested world that is constantly waging war against you. Even though you know in your mind and heart how to live and serve God, you still live in this world and the world ruthlessly competes for control over your life. That is why God sent Jesus. God knows and understands that we are born in sin and that it is impossible for us to live a sinless life without His intervention. But because of what Jesus has done for us when we truly repent, we will be forgiven over and over and over. The key, however, is that you *truly* repent. In doing so, you consciously change your direction and abandon your agenda.

➤ According to 2 Corinthians 7:9-10, what is the difference between godly sorrow and worldly sorrow?

List an example of each of these two types of sorrows in your own life.

Since the Holy Spirit dwells in your heart, you will feel an intense sorrow when you disobey God. God designed this sorrow to lead you toward repentance. You, however, can choose to ignore His prompting and walk in disobedience. God will not force you to obey, but He will allow you to feel sorrow until you acknowledge your disobedience and repent.

Though no one may ever know how you have sinned against God in your heart, the Holy Spirit knows. You may not be imprisoned, get cited or lose your reputation, but the heartache your sin inflicts is torture enough. In fact, until you repent, you will carry the burden and the consequences of that sin. As the Holy Spirit convicts you of sin, that conviction will continue to produce godly sorrow in you. When you truly repent and seek forgiveness, you can once again walk in freedom and experience God's peace and joy, never again to feel guilty for that sin.

>> If you are still tempted to feel guilty over your past sins, who is tempting and condemning you?

>> What does Romans 2:4 say about God's kindness?

>> What in your life have you felt convicted about and yet haven't dealt with? Do you need to confess something or turn away from something? Do you need to obey by doing something that the Holy Spirit is leading you to do?

Perhaps this is the first time you have heard of your need for repentance. Have you made the step of repentance in your life? Have you admitted your sin, turned around and begun to follow Jesus? Read John 3:16. Have you accepted God's love and accepted His Son, Jesus, as your Savior so that you have eternal life? If you want to learn more about this process, contact your First Place leader, your pastor or a trusted Christian friend who would be more than happy to lead you to redemption in Jesus Christ. Remember, He accepts you as you are right now and loves you immensely!

O God, may I never show contempt for the riches of Your kindness, tolerance and patience! Help me to realize that Your kindness leads me to repentance [see Romans 2:4].

Thank You, also, for godly sorrow that convicts me of my sin and leads me to repentance so that I may continue to walk in the light of Your presence. Thank You, Lord, that godly sorrow leaves absolutely no regret [see 2 Corinthians 7:9-10].

O Father, I love You and desire to walk with You and continually experience Your grace and presence.

DAY 3: *Sanctification*

At the moment of salvation you are sanctified, meaning you have been detached from the world and attached to God. You have been set apart; you are holy.

Sanctification is simply the journey—the process—of growing and maturing in your spiritual walk and level of intimacy with Jesus. As you study, trust and obey the Word of God, you will grow closer to Him; your relationship with Him will become more intimate and you will become more like Him. As you continue in this process, you will walk in the light of freedom and in Christ's victory.

➣ What do the following verses tell you about the process of sanctification?

Acts 26:18

Romans 15:16

1 Corinthians 1:2

1 Corinthians 6:9-11

⤳ What promise regarding the process of sanctification is found in 1 Thessalonians 5:23-24?

How does that promise give you hope?

Consider for a moment your commitment to the Live-It plan. No doubt it has taken great effort and discipline to walk the road toward a healthier lifestyle. Even though you may have had times of overindulgence, you continue to go back to your First Place meetings, receive encouragement from the group members, study the Word and walk forward rather than giving up or turning back. It is the same with the process of spiritual sanctification—it is an ongoing walk. Becoming sanctified is a daily, conscious effort. This is your identification with Christ. You have to die daily to your own fleshly desires in order to continue the process of being sanctified.

Examine your heart and life. Are you striving for the right things? Are you pursuing your own ambition or following the Lord's path? What is your agenda? How does it line up with God's? Sanctification has a price: It costs everything that is not of God.

I love You, Lord. Help me to rid myself of everything that is not of You. Help me to be willing to give it all up for the sake of righteousness.

Holy God, Thank You that You are faithful and will continue the process of sanctification in me so that my whole spirit, soul and body will be kept blameless [see 1 Thessalonians 5:23-24].

DAY 4: *Obedience*

Learning to obey God's commands regardless of how you feel is one of the most difficult processes of grace. But it is also absolutely necessary if you desire to be His child and to receive the blessings of His grace.

✎ What is the common thread in the following verses: John 14:15,23-24; 15:10-11; 1 John 5:2-3; 2 John 6?

What does this repetition tell you about the importance of obedience in your relationship to God?

We cannot claim to love God if we're not willing to put everything on the line for Him! Just the fact that you are doing a Bible study shows that you desire to grow closer and be more intimate with the Lord. That's a great place to start! You'll spend the rest of your life learning how to follow His commands and how to distinguish which attitudes befit His children.

✎ According to Micah 6:8, what does the Lord require of you?

Of the three commands, walking humbly is arguably the most difficult. But when we are truly humble before our awesome God, it is impossible to have a my-way-or-no-way attitude. Only when we are in our rightful place and attitude—humbly kneeling at His feet—will we desire to obey His commands. Humility before the Lord reminds us that He is God and we are not!

✎ As you read 1 Peter 2:13-15, what comes to mind when you think about submitting to someone else?

In 1 Peter 2:13, the Greek word *hupotasso* is translated "submit yourselves," meaning to subject one's self to the authority of another.[3] We are to submit ourselves to "every authority instituted among men." Submission is not synonymous with weakness, as our culture implies. Instead, it shows strength in your role as a bondservant—a willing slave—to Jesus Christ. When you submit to the authority of someone God has placed over you, you are submitting to Jesus Himself. There is no shame in that!

➺ Describe an area of your life in which you struggle to submit and/or obey.

Surrender that area to the Lord right now. Confess your heart attitude and ask the Holy Spirit to empower you to live righteously by submitting to authority in order to display a Christlike attitude and character.

 Lord, teach me to walk humbly with You and to obey Your commands, even when my sinful nature would rather do things my way.

Empower me by Your Holy Spirit to obey my earthly authorities—not only when their eyes are on me in order to win their favor but instead with sincerity of heart and reverence for You [see Colossians 3:22].

I praise You, Father, that I will receive Your inheritance as a reward, for it is the Lord Jesus Christ I am serving. In His name, amen [see Colossians 3:24].

DAY 5: *Prayer and Meditation*

After the process of grace begins in your life, it is critical to practice the discipline of prayer and daily meditation on the Word of God. While Bible study is a tool for learning God's truths, deeper growth will not occur without prayer and meditation on the lessons you will learn in His Word.

It is important to point out that the meditation you are to engage in is not an emptying of your mind, a practice many Eastern religions teach. Rather, it is a filling of your mind with God's truth and understanding how it applies to you. As you pray, don't use the time to merely give your to-do list to God. Instead, while forming a mental picture of the truth you've studied, ask the Lord to show you how best to apply it in your own life. While it is appropriate to cry out to God to meet your needs, He also wants you to engage in conversation with Him. He deeply desires to communicate His truths to you and to transform your life forever.

≫ According to Joshua 1:7-8, what does God command us to do?

What does He command us to *not* do?

What would be the results of obeying these commands?

≫ How do the following verses relate to meditating on God's Word? What are the benefits and results?

Psalm 1:2-3

Psalm 63:6-7

Psalm 119:12-16

Psalm 119:41-48

Psalm 119:97-105

The following is an example of how prayer and meditation on God's Word can be put into practice. As you read the following verse, begin to picture in your mind how this truth can affect your life and think of ways you can apply it personally.

[For my determined purpose is] that I may know Him [that I may progressively become more deeply and intimately acquainted with Him, perceiving and recognizing and understanding the wonders of His Person more strongly and more clearly], and that I may in the same way come to know the power outflowing from His resurrection [which it exerts over believers], and that I may so share His sufferings as to be continually transformed [in spirit into His likeness even] to His death (Philippians 3:10, AMP).

➣ What does it take to truly get to know another person?

In order to develop a personal, loving relationship with another person, you must spend time with him or her.

➣ Picture yourself living out Philippians 3:10. How does this Scripture apply to you?

As you cultivate your relationship with Christ, spending time with Him and getting to know Him better, He will reveal Himself, His power, His love and His grace to you. You will gain a greater understanding of His resurrection power. As you die to yourself, the same power that raised Jesus from the dead empowers you to experience Him, fight the battles and live victoriously. As you share in His sufferings, your life will never be the same. You will be continually changed and transformed forever.

Father God, I confess that my delight is in Your law, and I will meditate on it day and night [see Psalm 1:2].

Living Lord, draw near to me as I seek Your face through prayer and by meditating on You and Your written Word. My soul's deepest cry is to be intimately acquainted with You. Be merciful to Your servant and reveal Yourself to me!

DAY 6: *Reflections*

In this week's study, we looked at five steps to living in freedom. God's grace embodies each of these in order to fill your life with peace, hope and purpose. In order to fully identify with Christ, you must die to yourself daily. Have you identified areas in your life that must be put to death? You may grieve over giving up those things that grieve the heart of God; however, freedom will come as you acknowledge that it is impossible to fully enjoy something when you know you are being disobedient and that your disobedience is hindering an intimate, growing relationship with Jesus.

As you discern areas of disobedience, follow through with what is required of you today as the Holy Spirit reveals it. In place of the burden, Jesus will embrace you with His peace. Don't allow the enemy a stronghold. Allow the Holy Spirit to empower you to live a life of obedience and truth.

I know whom I have believed and am convinced that You, Lord, are able to guard what I have entrusted to You. I entrust this situation to You, Lord [see 2 Timothy 1:12].[4]

Lord, I do not want to be like those who refuse to pay attention to You. Please help me not turn my back in stubbornness and stop up my ears just because Your will is hard at times. Help me not make my heart as hard as flint and refuse to listen to the words that You, Lord Almighty, have sent by Your Spirit [see Zechariah 7:11-12].[5]

Lord God, cause my work to be produced by faith, my labor prompted by love and my endurance inspired by hope in my Lord Jesus Christ [see 1 Thessalonians 1:3].[6]

DAY 7: *Reflections*

This week's Scripture memory verse is a message to every believer that *everyone* needs Christ's redemption. Everyone must accept Him by faith and be justified and redeemed by His blood. Everything you have been given is because of His grace. The processes you've studied this week—acceptance, repentance, sanctification, obedience, and prayer and meditation—are gifts that He gives to enrich your relationship with Him. He longs for you to know Him. He loves you and celebrates you. Rest assured that He is constantly at work on your behalf.

The more time you spend in prayer and meditation on God's Word, the deeper and more intimate your relationship with Jesus will be. It can be difficult to discipline yourself to meditate on the Word when you are trying to juggle the responsibilities of your busy life. However, it is time well spent and is essential if you are to survive your busy and stressful lifestyle. Don't allow the cares of this world to choke out your time with your Father. In turn, you are promised a life filled with His peace, joy, comfort, strength and grace.

O God, speak to me so clearly through Your Word that I recognize Your voice. Help me to understand what You are making known to me, delighting me with Your Word so that I may celebrate with great joy [see Nehemiah 8:12].[7]

Guard my life and rescue me, O Lord. Let me not be put to shame, for I take refuge in You. May integrity and uprightness protect me, because my hope is in You [see Psalm 25:20-21].[8]

Father, I pray that You will cause no weapon forged against me to prevail. Enable me to refute the tongue of my accuser. Thank You for giving this heritage to Your servants, O Lord [see Isaiah 54:17].[9]

Notes

1. "NAS New Testament Greek Lexicon," *Crosswalk.com.* http://bible.crosswalk.com/Lexicons/Greek/grk.cgi?number=1205&version=nas (accessed June 24, 2003).
2. "KJV New Testament Greek Lexicon," *Crosswalk.com.* http://bible.crosswalk.com/Lexicons/Greek/grk.cgi?number=2112&version=kjv (accessed June 24, 2003).
3. "KJV New Testament Greek Lexicon," *Crosswalk.com.* http://bible.crosswalk.com/Lexicons/Greek/grk.cgi?number=5293&version=kjv (accessed September 9, 2003).
4. Beth Moore, *Praying God's Word* (Nashville, TN: Broadman and Holman, 2000), p. 231.
5. Ibid.

6. Ibid., p. 267.
7. Ibid.
8. Ibid., p. 318.
9. Ibid., p. 323.

GROUP PRAYER REQUESTS   TODAY'S DATE:_____

NAME	REQUEST	RESULTS

ATTITUDES OF GRACE

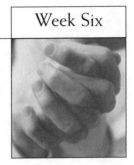

MEMORY VERSE

I am the vine; you are the branches. If a man remains in me and I in him, he will bear much fruit; apart from me you can do nothing.

John 15:5

Last week we learned about the processes of grace: acceptance, repentance, sanctification, obedience, and prayer and meditation. When we accept Jesus as our Savior, the lifelong process of becoming more like Him in our actions, thoughts and attitudes begins.

Have you ever heard the phrase "attitude is everything"? Our feelings and emotions largely dictate how we will act or react in any given situation. That's why developing a Christlike attitude is so important to your growth. Having a good attitude in unfavorable situations is difficult, but with Christ's strength and power we can! (see Philippians 4:13; Colossians 1:11).

In this week's study we are going to delve a little deeper into the attitudes we need to develop as we walk the road to sanctification. These attitudes are also called the fruit of the Spirit (see Galatians 5:22-23), because the Holy Spirit is the One who ultimately causes them to grow in us. This week's memory verse reminds us that the only way we can bear this fruit is by remaining in Christ.

DAY 1: *Love*

Galatians 5:22-23 gives us the list of the fruit of the Spirit. The first fruit listed is love.

➤ According to John 15:9-13, how do you remain in Jesus' love?

The command in verse 12 states that we are to love others as Christ loves us. What does a Christlike love for others entail?

Let's look at God's definition of true love.

> Love never gives up.
> Love cares more for others than for self.
> Love doesn't want what it doesn't have.
> Love doesn't strut,
> Doesn't have a swelled head,
> Doesn't force itself on others,
> Isn't always "me first,"
> Doesn't fly off the handle,
> Doesn't keep score of the sins of others,
> Doesn't revel when others grovel,
> Takes pleasure in the flowering of truth,
> Puts up with anything,
> Trusts God always,
> Always looks for the best,
> Never looks back,
> But keeps going to the end (1 Corinthians 13:4-7,
>   THE MESSAGE).

You may have heard this passage read in a wedding ceremony, but this actually describes Christ's love for you.

Read 1 Corinthians 13:4-7 again and circle three phrases that exemplify how Christ has shown His love to you.

Now look at those three phrases that you chose and think of someone to whom you need to demonstrate that kind of love. Write his or her initials next to the appropriate phrase.

A graceful, loving attitude shares the love of God with others. Who in your life is hard to love? How might you show godly love to that person this week?

One way to express love to others is by encouraging them. One of the Nine Commitments of First Place is to encourage others, especially other group members.

>> How will you express that commitment this week to one of your group members?

As you adopt an attitude of love toward others, you remain in Christ's love and will experience the joy that comes from watching the Holy Spirit transform your heart. There will obviously be times you fall short, but remember that developing an attitude of grace is a process. Don't give up!

O God, thank You for Your Son, Jesus. I thank You that He laid down His life for me. Father, I pray that I would have that same kind of love, that I would be willing to lay down my life for a friend [see John 15:13].

Lord, I pray that as Your Spirit develops an attitude of love in my heart, I would demonstrate that love not only with words but also through my actions [see 1 John 3:18].

Father God, give me a greater understanding and revelation of how much You love me, and with that understanding, empower me to love You.

DAY 2: *Joy and Peace*

As you abide in Christ's love and learn to extend it to others, His joy will be in you and your joy will be complete. When your attitude is in line with Christ's, the fruit of joy is a natural response and your attitude is full of His grace.

>> According to John 15:10-11, what is the key to experiencing Jesus' joy?

How would you define the kind of joy that only Jesus brings?

≫ Read James 1:2-4. Describe a time when you have experienced that kind of joy in spite of your circumstances.

≫ How can the "joy of the Lord" be your strength (Nehemiah 8:10)?

The peace of God is not a result of positive circumstances in your life—instead, it is a direct result of how you *respond* to circumstances in your life. As you look to Jesus Christ, you are able to experience peace and joy regardless of your circumstances. It is a supernatural work of God's Spirit in you, another awesome example of the power of God.

≫ According to Philippians 4:6-7, how do you obtain God's peace?

How would you define peace that "transcends all understanding"?

Not only does God's peace transcend all understanding, but it also guards your heart and your mind in Christ Jesus. If you have tough circumstances swirling all around you, God promises you His peace if you pray with thanksgiving. When you praise and thank the Lord—especially when you don't *feel* like it—He will calm your heart and mind, and you will begin to rest in His assurance. In addition to memorizing this week's

Scripture memory verse, also memorize Philippians 4:6-7 if you haven't already. Keep it close to your heart and meditate on it when you are overwhelmed.

> If you are missing out on God's peace and joy, ask the Holy Spirit to show you any areas in your life that you need to turn over to God and then trust Him to take care of them. Write down the areas that come to mind. Prayerfully turn these areas over to Him.

In the days ahead, as you offer up a sacrifice of praise and thanksgiving to God on a daily basis, regardless of your circumstances, you will be able to look back and see how God has brought you through by changing your attitude, your perspective and even your understanding of your situation.

Your weekly Commitment Record helps you keep track of your accomplishments each week; allow it to motivate you to continue striving toward a healthier lifestyle. If you have setbacks, don't be discouraged! Pray for God's strength and power to move forward once again. Rely on His strength alone to reach the goals you have set for yourself.

Father God, Your Word clearly says to not be anxious about anything but to present my requests to You. Fill me with Your peace—a peace that is beyond my understanding and that guards my heart and my mind from worry [see Philippians 4:6-7].

Thank You, O Lord, that I don't have to sorrow as the world does. I don't have to give in to fear or worry because my hope is in You! Fill my heart with Your praises and songs of thanksgiving as I go about my day.

DAY 3: *Patience, Kindness and Goodness*

The word translated "patience"—*makrothumia* in the Greek—can also be translated "long-suffering."[1] Long-suffering can be summed up in this way:

It is a quality of endurance and self-control in the face of stress, frustration, pain and/or sorrow.

➤ Second Corinthians 6:3-10 describes a wide variety of hardships that Paul and his fellow travelers had to endure. List the "negatives/hardships" and the "positives/fruit" of these experiences.

Negatives/Hardships   Positives/Fruit

➤ How might patience be a fruit of trials and difficulties?

While you may never suffer as Paul did, it is important that you allow your suffering and hardships to bring about godliness in your life. As unbelievers observe the fruit in your life in the midst of pain and suffering, they encounter the grace and the power of God and you become His salt and light in their dark world (see Matthew 5:13-16).

➤ According to Colossians 3:12, why are we to clothe ourselves with "compassion, kindness, humility, gentleness and patience"? How are these attitudes related?

We tend to use the words "kindness" and "goodness" interchangeably, but they have two distinct meanings. Kindness is an outward display of benevolence but does not necessarily reflect a person's inner character. It is expressed in deeds carried out with grace. Even nonbelievers can show kindness to others. Goodness, however, is the display of moral character by a believer who has been transformed by God's power and holiness.

➤ Read the story of the "woman who had lived a sinful life" in Luke 7:36-50. What did the woman do for Jesus?

What upset the Pharisee about the situation (v. 39)?

What lesson did Jesus teach in response to the Pharisee's attitude (vv. 40-47)?

Acting in kindness often requires us to go out of our way to help another person or to do something that is humbling. We might be called to step out of our comfort zone to show kindness to someone.

➤ Ephesians 5:8-11 contrasts goodness with the darkness of the world and warns that we are to "have nothing to do with the fruitless deeds of darkness, but rather expose them." What are examples of the deeds of darkness in our world and how might Christians expose them?

Jesus exemplified kindness and goodness throughout the Gospels by loving people, touching their lives and healing their minds, hearts and bodies.

➤ During the week ahead, ask the Lord to show you ways to demonstrate the attitudes of kindness and goodness to others. In your Prayer Journal, record any experiences that you might have.

Father God, as Your chosen one, help me to daily clothe myself with compassion, kindness, humility, gentleness and patience [see Colossians 3:12].

Lord, I know that doing kind things for others means nothing if my heart harbors impure motives. Change me from the inside out so that my kind deeds are a natural outpouring of a pure and righteous heart.

DAY 4: *Faithfulness*

The Bible is filled with references to God's faithfulness toward His people. "Know therefore that the Lord your God . . . is the faithful God, keeping his covenant of love to a thousand generations of those who love him and keep his commands" (Deuteronomy 7:9). Just as He does with the other fruit of the Spirit, God expects us to demonstrate faithfulness in our lives and actions.

➤ According to Matthew 25:14-30, what did the master say to *and* do for the two servants who were faithful stewards of their talents?

Why didn't the third servant increase his one talent?

Are you afraid of God? You needn't be; He is a trustworthy, loving God who has your best interests at heart. Are you struggling to keep the Nine Commitments of First Place? He desires the best for you and will help you to faithfully follow through on these commitments.

➤ In what ways are the following verses an encouragement to you as you struggle to keep your commitments?

1 Corinthians 1:7-9

1 Corinthians 10:13

Philippians 1:6

1 Thessalonians 5:23-24

Can you believe that? God has promised to help you perfect you! Do you trust Him to accomplish His purposes in your life? Can you trust your trustworthy Father?

Father, Your Word has promised that You will be faithful to help me be faithful. Thank You for Your awesome love that wants only the best for me. Help me today to faithfully obey Your will for my life and to keep my First Place commitments.

DAY 5: *Gentleness and Self-Control*

Our society does not honor gentleness, even to the point of considering it a sign of weakness. Yet in Matthew 11:29, Jesus describes Himself as "gentle and humble in heart." He certainly was not weak, standing up to the religious leaders of the day who were leading people astray and withstanding the cruelty and brutality of his trials and physical punishments.

In his second letter to the church at Corinth, Paul showed that gentleness does not keep us from being bold when the occasion arises.

≫ According to 2 Corinthians 10:1-2, what circumstances would cause Paul to become bold?

≫ Describe a time when you had to mix gentleness with boldness to confront someone.

How did Jesus display His faithfulness to you during this time?

The fact that you are in the First Place program shows that you desire to develop or to better exercise self-control. This precious attitude of grace impacts every area of your life, from food and exercise to our thought patterns, from controlling our tongue to sexual purity.

➣ According to 1 Corinthians 6:12-13, what is the essence of self-control?

➣ We are all tempted by things that are permissible but that are not God's best for us. With what permissible things do you struggle most?

➣ In 1 Corinthians 10:13, what has God promised to do for us when we struggle with temptation?

Jesus was the ultimate example of gentleness and self-control. When you follow Him and take on His yoke, He teaches you what it means to be gentle and self-controlled in every area of your life. As you submit your heart to these attitudes of grace, you will watch your life be transformed through the Holy Spirit.

O God, make my heart tender and gentle, like that of Your Son, Jesus Christ. Teach me to be like Him, even in the face of persecution.

Father, I want every area of my life to be in control today—from my thoughts to what I eat. Give me the strength necessary to say no to those things that are not beneficial to me.

I praise You, Father, that You who began a good work in me will carry it on to completion until the day of Christ Jesus [see Philippians 1:6].

DAY 6: *Reflections*

In this week's study we have focused on developing an attitude of grace no matter the circumstances. It is during times of testing that others can see the difference Christ is making in your life. As you obey God, remain in His love and desperately depend on Him, you will be immersed in His love, peace and joy—and others will have an encounter with grace when they witness His grace at work in your life.

During times of hardship, it can be tempting to ask yourself, *Why is this happening to me?* As hard as suffering is, it can cause you to run to Jesus and depend on Him like nothing else. When life is going smoothly, it can be easy to forget that the privileges you have and the prosperity you enjoy are gifts from God. You can fool yourself into believing that the things you enjoy are the result of your hard work and determination. When you buy into this deceptive thinking, you forget that not only is everything you have a gift from God but that your life itself is also a gift. Through hardships, we are reminded that God is our strength and our refuge (see Psalm 46:1) and that there is nothing certain in this world but Him.

Lord, though I have not seen You, I want to love You deeply; and even though I do not see You now, I want to believe in You and be filled with an inexpressible and glorious joy [see 1 Peter 1:8].[2]

Father God, help me to be self-controlled and alert. My enemy the devil prowls around like a roaring lion looking for someone to devour. Help me to resist him, standing firm in the faith. I can be assured that other believers throughout the world are undergoing the same kind of sufferings [see 1 Peter 5:8-9].[3]

God, as one of Your chosen people, holy and dearly loved, help me to clothe myself with compassion, kindness, humility, gentleness and patience [see Colossians 3:12].[4]

DAY 7: *Reflections*

The keys to bearing fruit are remaining in Christ's love and obeying His commands. But what happens when it seems as though God doesn't answer your prayers even when you are remaining faithful? Do you feel that He is failing you? One of the greatest things that you can know from your trials is how good God is and how much He loves you. Though circumstances may not change, God is absolutely at work in the midst of your difficulty. Just as a loving earthly father knows that not everything his children ask for is good for them, so does God know what is best for you. He *does* answer every prayer, but sometimes His answer is no or not yet. Wait patiently and have faith in His wisdom, knowing that the difficult times are times of growth.

Allow trials and hardships to be pivotal points in your life. As you trust Him and endure until the answer comes, His faithfulness will be displayed above and beyond anything you could ever imagine. If you are still skeptical or feel weak under your heavy burden, begin asking God to soften and strengthen your heart. Confess that you are having a hard time believing and trusting Him right now in the midst of your trial. Ask Him for a greater measure of faith. In faith offer up a sacrifice of praise and thanksgiving every time you think about your burden. Read the Psalms for examples of praise in the midst of intense hardship.

God, You know the way that I take; when You have tested me, I will come forth as gold. My feet will closely follow Your steps; I desire to keep to Your way without turning aside. I desire never to depart from the commands of Your lips. Cause me to treasure the words of Your mouth more than my daily bread [see Job 23:10-12].[5]

My Father, please help me to be on my guard; stand firm in the faith; be a person of courage; be strong; and to do everything in love [see 1 Corinthians 16:13].[6]

O Lord, help me to continue to grow the fruit of the Spirit—love, joy, peace, patience, kindness, goodness, faithfulness, gentleness and self-control [see Galatians 5:22-23]. When I struggle, remind me that You have promised to help me to have the attitude of Christ.

Notes

1. "KJV New Testament Greek Lexicon," *Crosswalk.com*. http://bible.crosswalk.com/Lexicons/Greek /grk.cgi?number=3115&version=kjv (accessed June 27, 2003).
2. Beth Moore, *Praying God's Word* (Nashville, TN: Broadman and Holman, 2000) p. 44.
3. Ibid., p. 55.
4. Ibid., p. 68.
5. Ibid., p. 215.
6. Ibid., p. 327.

GROUP PRAYER REQUESTS TODAY'S DATE:_____

NAME	REQUEST	RESULTS

KNOWING THE GOD OF ALL GRACE

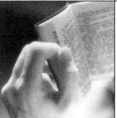

MEMORY VERSE
The name of the LORD is a strong tower;
the righteous run to it and are safe.
Proverbs 18:10

Do you realize that as a believer, the same presence and power that protected and led the Israelites, the same presence and power that raised Jesus from the dead, lives inside you? It's wonderfully true! And that same God loves you so much that He chooses to reveal Himself—His nature—to you. When the Israelites caught a glimpse of God's character, they responded by calling Him by a name that reflected the characteristic He displayed.

In this week's study we will learn more about the God of all grace as we explore some of the names that the Israelites attributed to Him.

DAY 1: Jehovah-Shammah—*The Lord Is There*

Ezekiel 48:35 describes the city of Jerusalem as Yahweh-Shammah "THE LORD IS THERE."[1] ("Yahweh" is the Hebrew transliteration of the word that we translate "Jehovah.") This name speaks of God's personal involvement in our lives.

➤ How does Psalm 23 point out God's personal involvement in our lives?

➤ Psalm 139:7-10 describes another aspect of the Lord's personal involvement in our lives. How does the fact that you cannot hide from God affect your relationship with Him?

✎ What is the promise of Joshua 1:5? Do you believe God's promise?

If not, what keeps you from accepting it?

If you are struggling with accepting and believing the truth about Jehovah-Shammah, "the Lord is there," call out to Him right now. Ask Him to make His presence known to you. Whenever you are feeling depressed, lonely or discouraged, call upon the name of Jehovah-Shammah, believing He is right there with you. At the same time, if you are exhilarated about something that God has blessed you with, call out to Jehovah-Shammah, praising Him for His blessings and presence. Your God is there with you always. Praise Him!

O Jehovah-Shammah, where can I go from Your spirit? Where can I flee from Your presence? If I go up to the heavens, You are there. If I make my bed in the depths, You are there. If I rise on the wings of the dawn, if I settle on the far side of the sea, even there Your hand will guide me, Your right hand will hold me fast [see Psalm 139:7-10].

You, my Lord, have never forsaken those who seek You. I thank You that You are always here with me and will never leave me nor forsake me [see Joshua 1:5].

Thank You that I can call upon You, Jehovah-Shammah, whenever I am feeling lonely or hurting. I praise You, O God, that You are here with me!

DAY 2: El Roi—*The God Who Sees*

No matter what you go through, there is nothing in your life hidden from "the God who sees." You can take comfort knowing you are never alone and that God knows what you are facing and wants to help you succeed.

Genesis 16:1-15 tells the story of a slave woman named Hagar and the selfishness of her mistress Sarai. Although God had promised a son to Abram through Sarai, Sarai had become impatient waiting for God to fulfill His promise and had given Hagar to Abram so that Hagar might have his child. When Hagar became pregnant, Sarai mistreated her and she ran away.

➢ According to Genesis 16:7, where was Hagar when the Lord spoke to her through the angel?

➢ How did Hagar address God (vv. 13-14)?

Hagar realized that no matter where she went or in what circumstances she found herself, God saw her and cared about her.

➢ How does it make you feel to know that God was there and saw everything that had happened to Hagar?

➢ What instruction was given to Hagar by the angel, and what would be the result of her obedience (vv. 9-10)?

If you have been mistreated or abused by someone, God wants to heal your wounded heart. You don't have to carry the burden of someone's sin against you any longer. Through God, you can let go of your painful past and be released from the chains of suffering that have held you prisoner. God desires—and is able—to heal your heart. He has seen you and heard your cries. Take the matter to God in thoughtful prayer and ask Him to direct your path and help you to let go.[2]

Look at one more incredible passage today; read Psalm 139:15-16. Even before you were conceived, God knew you!

➤ Whether you are grateful beyond expression or still struggling with anger, heartache, pain and confusion, express your feelings to El Roi, "the God who sees," in a prayer.

Now proclaim the truth of God's Word by faith and allow it to minister to and comfort your spirit. God is continually at work. Ask Him for an even greater measure of faith to trust Him.

El Roi, You see everything, including the secret sins I hold in my heart. Make my heart clean, Lord God, that what You see will be pleasing in Your sight.

I praise You, El Roi, that when I was woven together in the depths of the earth, Your eyes saw my unformed body. You know every intricate detail about me! I trust that You have a plan for every day of my life, because You saw every single one of them before they came to be [see Psalm 139:15-16].

DAY 3: Jehovah-Rophi—*The Lord Who Heals*

As living beings on this earth, we cannot escape the physical effects sin has had on our world. But thanks be to God, Jehovah-Rophi, "the Lord who heals," who stands ready to heal us.

➤ According to 2 Chronicles 7:14, what four things do God's people need to do in order to have their land forgiven and healed?

How can you apply this verse to your own life?

⇒ According to Psalm 147:3, what does the Lord do?

What has broken your heart or wounded you? How do you need Jehovah Rophi to heal you?

⇒ How did Jesus heal Peter's mother-in-law in Matthew 8:14? Where you do you need His touch in your life?

⇒ According to 1 Peter 2:24, by what means have you been healed?

When you accepted Jesus into your life, you were instantly spiritually healed. Your sins were forgiven, your slate was wiped clean, and your debt was erased. Spiritual healing is often the first step in healing the other areas of your life: mental, emotional and physical.

Unlike spiritual healing, physical and emotional healing don't always come instantly. Don't let this discourage you! The Lord supplies everything you need on this earth (see Philippians 4:19), and continuing physical or emotional health problems are not evidence that He has deserted you. On the contrary, He is always with you, and He wants to help you live a full life despite any health concerns you face.

When you follow through with the commitments you made when you joined First Place, you will experience life-changing transformation, including in your physical well-being. While you may continue to suffer from diabetes, high blood pressure or other particular problems, your overall health will improve—and as your spiritual, emotional and overall physical health improve, it will be easier to deal with areas in which you need healing.

As you memorize Scripture, read and study your Bible, spend time in prayer each day, encourage others, attend your First Place meetings and are diligent in filling out your CRs, God will be at work in all areas of your life to transform you into the person He has called you to be.

Thank You, Jehovah-Rophi, for healing my greatest ailment—spiritual separation from You. Jesus, You bore my sins in Your body on the cross, that I might die to sin and live to righteousness. It is only by Your wounds that I am truly healed [see 1 Peter 2:24].

O God, I confess that I need You! I thank You that You are the Lord who heals—Jehovah-Rophi—I need healing in these areas: [state areas]. I ask in faith, knowing that Your timing is perfect and Your plan for me is good.

DAY 4: Jehovah-Jireh—*The Lord Will Provide*

When you read the story of Abraham's devotion to the Lord in Genesis 22—even to the point of willingness to offer his son Isaac as a sacrifice—it is not hard to imagine how heart wrenching that must have been for Abraham, particularly when Isaac asked his father where the animal for the burnt offering was.

⇛ In Genesis 22:7-8, how did Abraham answer Isaac's question?

⇛ In Genesis 17:21, what promise had God made to Abraham, and how do you think this promise gave Abraham hope when he prepared to sacrifice Isaac?

❧ Have you ever been given a promise by God and had to wait for the fulfillment of that promise (or perhaps you are still waiting)? What kept you (or keeps you) hoping and believing in that promise?

❧ According to Genesis 22:13, God provided the ram in the thicket as the sacrificial offering. What did Abraham name that place on the mountain?

❧ In Genesis 22:2,12,16, how did the Lord refer to Abraham's son? What is the significance of this?

The story of Abraham and Isaac foreshadows the story of Jesus. Consider John 1:29—like the ram in the thicket, God provided His only Son as the sacrifice to take away the sins of the world. Look at John 3:16—like Abraham, our Jehovah-Jireh didn't hold back anything when He provided His Son as *the* way for us to be eternally His.

❧ In light of what Jehovah-Jireh did for you through the sacrifice of His Son, does this change how you feel about God's ultimately fulfilling every promise He has made to you? Please explain.

❧ Is there a need in your life that is so pressing that you have nowhere to turn but to the Lord your God? Please explain.

Cry out to Jehovah-Jireh today for His provision. Offer up your praise and thanksgiving in the midst of your struggle or hardship. God is there with you. He sees, He heals and He provides. Praise Him!

 O God, thank You for providing a way for me to have eternal life. Thank You, Jehovah-Jireh, for not sparing Your only Son, in order that I might be free from sin's power. I know that You will also generously provide everything I need [see Romans 8:32].

I praise You, Jehovah-Jireh, that You will meet all my needs according to Your glorious riches in Christ Jesus [see Philippians 4:19].

DAY 5: *Our God*

Today, we're going to recap some of the ways the Word describes grace and how grace relates to God's many different names.

➢ As you read each of the following Scripture passages, ask the Holy Spirit to show you what He wants to teach you through them. Ask God to open your heart and for understanding. Write down what you hear Him speaking to you. Please take your time. As you read, think about your study this week and how knowing the names of God has impacted your understanding of His grace.

Luke 2:40

John 1:14,16-17

Acts 15:11

1 Corinthians 1:4

Ephesians 4:7

Philippians 1:7

2 Thessalonians 2:16; 3:16

Is there a particular verse that you felt spoke especially to you today? Please explain.

⟫ Which name of God ministered to you the most this week?

☐ Jehovah-Shammah   ☐ Jehovah-Rophi
☐ El-Roi   ☐ Jehovah-Jireh

All that you have, all that you are, all that you will ever be is all by God's grace. Your eternal destiny is sealed in Christ Jesus, bought and paid for by His blood. God's grace has made you free and victorious.

Father God, thank You for lavishing Your grace on me. By the fullness of Your grace I have received one blessing after another [see John 1:16].

Thank You that Your greatest blessings are intangible: Your provision, presence, watchfulness, healing and salvation. Continue to show me glimpses of Yourself, Lord God, as I continue to grow in the grace and knowledge of You. To You be the glory both now and forever! [see 2 Peter 3:18].

DAY 6: *Reflections*

While studying God's awesome names and character, it's hard to not become overwhelmed with His presence.

Whatever obstacle you are facing, call out to the One who is there, to the One who sees, to the One who heals, to the One who provides. His deepest desire is for you to know and trust Him. Allow Him to use every circumstance in your life to deepen your relationship with Him. As you surrender and are desperately dependent on Him, He will reveal Himself in ways you could never imagine. What the enemy means for harm and pain in your life, God will turn into a blessing.

Yours, my Lord, is the greatness and the power and the glory and the majesty and the splendor, for everything in heaven and earth is Yours. Yours, my own heavenly Father, is the kingdom, and You are exalted as head above all [see 1 Chronicles 29:11].[3]

My Father, Your kingdom is an everlasting kingdom, and Your dominion endures throughout all generations. You, my Lord, are faithful to all Your promises and loving toward all You have made [see Psalm 145:13].[4]

Many, O Lord my God, are the wonders you have done. The things you planned for us no one can recount to you; were I to speak and tell of them, they would be too many to declare [Psalm 40:5].

DAY 7: *Reflections*

This week's memory verse speaks volumes and ministers comfort to the brokenhearted and wounded. Continue to cry out to God for personal revelation of His freedom through His awesome grace and character.

The meanings and impact of the names of God bring another dynamic into your relationship with Him. The Lord isn't off in the distance somewhere, watching from afar as you deal with life; rather, He is constantly at work and is faithful to bring you through your trials stronger and healthier than before. His names stand as a reminder of how in love He is with you and how involved He is in every aspect of your life. He so desires that you know Him. He will use everything that happens in your life for His glory and purpose. As you trust in and desperately depend on Him, your life will continue to grow and change. Allow the Lord to mold and shape you. As you respond obediently during times of rejoicing and times of trial, you'll continue to gain wisdom and insight into the person and character of God.

You, my God, are the Rock. Your works are perfect, and all Your ways are just. You are a faithful God who does no wrong. You are upright and just [see Deuteronomy 32:4].[5]

You alone are my rock and my salvation; You are my fortress, I will not be shaken. My salvation and my honor depend on You; You are my mighty rock, my refuge [see Psalm 62:6-7].[6]

Lord, please help me to revere Your name. You have promised that if I do, the sun of righteousness will rise with healing in its wings and that I will go out and leap like a calf released from the stall [see Malachi 4:2].[7]

Notes

1. Kenneth Barker, gen. ed., *The NIV Study Bible* (Grand Rapids, MI: Zondervan Publishing House, 1995), p. 1288.
2. If you are carrying the burden of past abuse, seek counseling from your pastor or a Christian counselor. Often we need the help of an outsider to see the best way to put a situation to rest. As always, test the counsel you are given against the Word of God. In this way, you will know how to proceed on your path toward freedom. May the peace and joy of the Lord be abundant in your heart!
3. Beth Moore, *Praying God's Word* (Nashville, TN: Broadman and Holman, 2000), p. 23.
4. Ibid.
5. Ibid., p. 29.
6. Ibid.
7. Ibid.

GROUP PRAYER REQUESTS   TODAY'S DATE:_____

NAME	REQUEST	RESULTS

GRACE-FILLED MEN AND WOMEN

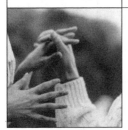

MEMORY VERSE

So then, just as you received Christ Jesus as Lord, continue to live in him, rooted and built up in him, strengthened in the faith as you were taught, and overflowing with thankfulness.

Colossians 2:6-7

There are countless men and women throughout history who undeniably lived grace-filled lives. What did these people possess that you can't? *Nothing.* Every single one of these people was imperfect—just like you and me, and you can successfully live a grace-filled life too.

In this week's study, we're going to take a look at five men and women from the Bible who demonstrated grace. As you learn about them, allow their stories to encourage you. Soak in God's truth this week, and continue to pray for the process of transforming your life.

DAY 1: *Humility*

In week six we read the story about the woman "who had lived a sinful life" (Luke 7:37) and how she humbled herself by doing the unthinkable: She approached Jesus at the Pharisee's house and washed His feet with her tears and an expensive bottle of perfume. Although we don't know the name of this woman, her humility before Jesus so impacted Him that her story has been recorded in the Bible. Because of her willingness to come before the Lord in humility, Jesus said to her, "Your sins are forgiven" (v. 48). Be mindful today about your own heart and what Jesus has done for you.

➺ Reread the story of the sinful woman in Luke 7:36-50. What is it about this woman that stands out to you?

This woman pursued Jesus to honor and serve Him. She didn't come upon Him by accident; she sought Him out. There was a chance He would reject her, yet she went anyway. When she found Him, the woman began to weep over her unworthiness (v. 38). In her brokenness, she displayed extreme love, humility and reverence for Jesus.

In verse 47, what did Jesus say about the woman's many sins?

What was the reason Jesus forgave the woman and instructed her to "go in peace" (v. 50)?

Jesus told a parable describing two men who owed different amounts of money (vv. 40-43). When the moneylender canceled both debts, the man who had owed more was more ecstatic over the news. Because he had been forgiven more, he loved the moneylender more than the other man did.

You have been forgiven a debt far greater than the man who owed 500 denarii! How should this knowledge move your heart toward humility?

This humble woman exemplified the fear of the Lord. Regardless of what anyone said or thought, she wanted to be where Jesus was, to bless, honor and worship Him. As a result, she received and experienced His grace.

You can also experience the grace of God when you humble yourself before Him.

O Father God, I bow at Your feet to worship You. I praise You and thank You for forgiving me and setting me free.

Lord, as I humble my heart before You, teach me Your ways and what is right in Your eyes [see Psalm 25:9].

Thank You for teaching me humility through this incredible woman, Lord. May You look at me with such favor and bless me with Your approval.

DAY 2: *Loyalty*

In today's study, let's take a look at a wise and loyal woman named Abigail. This woman's quick action saved her husband, Nabal, from being killed by David, even though Nabal deserved David's wrath. Abigail's loyalty did not go unnoticed by David. As you learn about Abigail today, think about your own life and cry out to God for His wisdom and knowledge to guide you through circumstances you face.

➤ Read Abigail's story in 1 Samuel 25. What is it about Abigail that stands out to you the most?

Abigail somehow saw the big picture. Though Nabal was rude and mean-spirited, she knew that it would not be right for David to avenge himself and kill her husband. Abigail was articulate and sensible in dealing with what her husband had done, and she was even willing to take the blame for his actions. She was a loyal wife—and loyal to God. She knew that God would deal with Nabal in His own timing. And He did (vv. 37-38).

➤ According to 1 Samuel 25:28-29, what did Abigail say the Lord would do for David?

What was the reason the Lord would do these things for David?

➤ Have you faced the temptation to seek revenge against someone? What usually happens when we seek personal revenge?

Romans 12:17 reminds us that we are not to "repay anyone evil for evil" and that we need to be "careful to do what is right." Doing what is right is not always the most appealing thing to do. It must have been very hard for Abigail to go to David to beg his mercy on her less-than-loving husband, but she chose to do the right thing and God did not fail to take notice.

➤ How did Abigail's character express grace?

➤ According to 1 Samuel 25:39, how did God honor Abigail?

God always honors obedience. Sometimes our judgment is clouded by anger, bitterness or disappointment, but He will provide a way for us to obey Him. Give your decisions to Him, and ask for His grace and for Him to help you choose what is right in His sight.

Father God, thank You for Your salvation and the wisdom that comes from it. I praise You for Your Word and the example it sets before me.

Help me to repay evil with good. Heal my heart, O God, and help me forgive those who have hurt me. Help me to focus on You and the freedom that comes through Jesus [see Romans 12:17].

Precious Jesus, You were loyal to Your Father to the point of death. Teach me that loyalty—that I might die to ungraciousness daily.

DAY 3: *Forgiveness*

The entire Old Testament is the story of God's grace and forgiveness toward Israel. He compared His Chosen People numerous times to an unfaithful wife. God chose to use His prophet Hosea to be a living example of that grace, turning his life into a metaphor of God's dealings with Israel.

➤ In Hosea 1:2-9, what did God call Hosea to do?

If this were the end of the story, we might smile and think, *How sweet!* Hosea showed more grace in marrying Gomer than many of us would ever dream of. But this isn't the end of the story. This godly man would show even more character in the remainder of the story.

Hosea 3 tells that despite Hosea's grace in marrying Gomer, she went back to her life as a prostitute. She repaid his generosity and care with a humiliating slap in the face. I don't think any of us would have blamed Hosea had he washed his hands of her at this point! He in fact had every right to have her stoned as an adulteress.

➤ According to 3:2, what did Hosea do in response to Gomer's abandonment?

Read verse 3. Not only did Hosea purchase his unfaithful wife's freedom, but he also took her back to his own household and gave her yet another chance. The level of forgiveness Hosea displayed toward Gomer is unfathomable by the world, but as Christians we've been introduced to a grace and forgiveness a thousand times greater! Because God has forgiven us a debt that far surpasses that of an adulterous wife, we are free to forgive even the most grievous of offenses committed against us.

➤ Think of the one person in your life whom you have had the most difficulty forgiving. What did he or she do to offend you (without mentioning names)?

How does this person's offense toward you compare with what God has forgiven you for?

Hosea is an incredible example of a man who displayed grace. His dealings with his wife are an example to all of us. But don't forget: None of these grace-filled men and women possess qualities that you cannot attain with the Lord's help! You can display abundant grace and forgiveness like Hosea did because you can go to the same source—the God of all grace.

Dear Lord, thank You for the abundant grace and forgiveness You show me daily. By the world's standards, You should have given up on me long ago! And yet, Your compassions are new every morning. Great is Your faithfulness! [see Lamentations 3:22-23].

Thank You, Father, for empowering Hosea to love and forgive an adulterous woman, for it serves as a vivid example of how I need to show grace to others. Empower me to go and do likewise.

DAY 4: *Faithfulness*

The story of Hannah is an amazing telling of pain, faith, love, commitment, vows and miracles. Hannah experienced it all. And through it all, she remained faithful to her word. She obediently followed through with her vow to God and, as a result, was blessed immeasurably.

➤ As you read 1 Samuel 1—2:21, what is it about Hannah that stands out to you the most?

➤ What was the result of Hannah's vow and commitment?

How did God bless her after she followed through with her commitment?

What Hannah did may be unfathomable to the world, but what a testimony of commitment and obedience!

➤ What does Matthew 5:33-37 say about the importance of keeping your word?

What is the source of broken oaths or commitments?

➤ What commitments have you made that you haven't followed through with yet?

➤ What is hindering you from remaining true to your word?

Elkanah loved Hannah even when she didn't have children. He was always concerned for her when she was sad and depressed about being barren. She was more valuable to him than his other wife, who bore him several children. He loved Hannah.

This is another example of Christ's love for you. Hannah was honored and loved by her husband. Elkanah knew that she prayed and worshiped God. He later honored her decision to give Samuel to the Lord—after all, Samuel was his son too! She remained true to her word, and God honored her faithfulness by blessing her with more children. God opened her womb.

➤ In what ways do you identify with Hannah?

➤ Describe how Hannah's character expresses God's grace.

Part of the success of your involvement in First Place depends on keeping the Nine Commitments. What commitments are you not fully following? Ask the Lord to empower you by the Holy Spirit to keep your commitments—whether they be your First Place commitments or your commitments to others or even to God Himself. This is between you and God. Pursue what it takes to remain in an intimate, abiding relationship with Him.

Remember that God gives you the grace and the power to obey. Your freedom is at stake. Fight for your freedom. Don't allow the enemy a foothold by convincing yourself that keeping your commitments is not a big deal. If you are obedient, God works out all the details. Your obedience to God is more important than what anyone else might think.

 Father, I pray that my yes would be yes and my no would be no. I pray that the words of my mouth would not be spoken carelessly but be spoken with thoughtfulness and purpose [see Matthew 5:37].

Lord, I ask for Your forgiveness for the times I've broken my word to You. Thank You for loving me and cleansing me from all unrighteousness [see 1 John 1:9].

DAY 5: *Integrity*

Today you'll learn about a man who in his youth was prideful and arrogant, hated by his brothers, sold into slavery and later in his life had an opportunity to experience and extend forgiveness and reconciliation. If you haven't guessed already, it is Joseph. God had a specific plan for Joseph's life from the very beginning. God tested him and allowed him to experience years of tremendous hardship; yet through it all, Joseph remained faithful to God and maintained his integrity as he lived as a slave and even endured prison. He humbled himself before the Lord, and as a result God blessed him greatly.

➤ Read Genesis 37:1-36; 45:1-8. What is it about Joseph that stands out to you the most?

In Genesis 39, God caused Joseph to find favor with Potiphar, who eventually made Joseph the head of his house. What followed next was an incredible testing of Joseph's integrity (see Genesis 39:6-12).

➣ According to verse 9, why wouldn't Joseph give in to the advances of Potiphar's wife?

Joseph's integrity got him thrown in prison because Potiphar's wife falsely accused him. Although it might not seem like it, God honored Joseph's integrity and used his prison experience for His ultimate good. Genesis 40—41:49 tell the intricate story of how Joseph came to find favor in Pharaoh's eyes and subsequently saved all of Egypt from starvation.

➣ Has there ever been a time when your integrity resulted in a negative reaction?

How did God bless you as a result of your willingness to be true to Him?

Read Genesis 41:50-52. Before Joseph even saw his brothers again, God had already enabled Joseph to forget his troubles and all the pain his brothers had caused him.

All that Joseph had experienced and endured was part of God's plan— and Joseph understood that. God was in control of every circumstance that came his way. Joseph could have harbored anger and bitterness toward his brothers and toward God for allowing him to suffer the way he did, but instead he forgave his brothers because he knew and trusted God. He continually humbled himself and desperately depended on God through it all. Joseph was faithful and obedient as God fulfilled the dreams he had had when he was a teenager. Joseph was a man of integrity and God honored him for that.

➤ How do you identify with Joseph?

➤ Describe how Joseph's character expresses grace.

In what ways would you like your heart to exemplify Christ's heart as Joseph's did?

Your protection is spread over those who love Your name. For surely, O Lord, You bless the righteous; You surround them with Your favor as with a shield [see Psalm 5:11-12].

May integrity and uprightness protect me because my hope is in You [see Psalm 25:21].

Father, help me hold fast to my integrity even when the outcome appears negative. I know and trust that You reward obedience with blessing, just as You blessed Your servant Joseph.

DAY 6: *Reflections*

In this week's study, we discovered the different ways men and women of the Bible have displayed grace in their lives. What an example they are to us today!

The woman who washed Jesus' feet with her tears and her hair recognized her position in Christ with humility. She understood how unworthy she was and what He had done for her. And as a result, she pursued Him with all her heart. Abigail exercised good, sound judgment. Hosea displayed incredible forgiveness. Hannah followed through with her vow to the Lord and gave her son to His service. Joseph was honored and greatly blessed by God for his integrity.

Each of these men and women demonstrated commitment. When you joined First Place, you made nine commitments. One of those commitments was to encourage others. Keep your commitment to do this and watch how giving and receiving encouragement and support can change your life and the lives of others.

Mighty God, help me to understand that I've been called by You to walk by faith and not by sight [see 2 Corinthians 5:7].[1]

Father God, Your Word tells me to know assuredly that You, the Lord, have set apart the godly for Yourself; You, Lord, will hear when I call to You [see Psalm 4:3].[2]

By faith Abraham, when called to go to a place he would later receive as his inheritance, obeyed and went, even though he did not know where he was going. Lord, help me to be willing to follow You in obedience even when I'm not sure where I'm heading [see Hebrews 11:8].[3]

DAY 7: *Reflections*

The memory verse this week exhorts you to remain steadfast and not grow weary in your daily walk with the Lord. Press on and continue to desperately depend on Him as you live your life. Don't allow the cares of this world to put out the flame of passion in your heart for Jesus. Remember the woman you studied in Day 1: Out of her understanding of who Jesus was came a deep reverence and awe for Him. Worshiping Jesus became her priority and she was not daunted by the conventions of the culture. The things of this world took a backseat to her desire to worship Jesus.

You may feel that you could never measure up to the men and women you have studied this week; however, because of the Holy Spirit living in you, You can serve and obey God in the same way they did. The Holy Spirit lives out these characteristics of grace in your life when you allow Him to do so. As you continue to grow in Christ, you will be built up by Him.

As we complete this week's study, let's focus on the last phrase of the Scripture memory verse: "overflowing with thankfulness." As you watch the Lord transform you in His grace, let your lips overflow with praises to Him! Rejoice over even the smallest victory, because it is evidence that the Holy Spirit is at work in your heart.

 Lord, because You are my help, I sing in the shadow of Your wings. My soul clings to You; Your right hand upholds me [see Psalm 63:7-8].[4]

O God, speak to me so clearly through Your Word that I recognize Your voice. Help me to understand what You are making known to me, delighting me with Your Word so that I may celebrate with great joy! [see Nehemiah 8:12].[5]

Lord, help me to keep my eyes looking straight ahead and fix my gaze directly before me. Make level paths for my feet and strengthen me to take only the ways that are firm. Help me not to swerve to the right or the left; keep my feet from evil [see Proverbs 4:25-27].[6]

Notes

1. Beth Moore, *Praying God's Word* (Nashville, TN: Broadman and Holman, 2000), p. 49.
2. Ibid., p. 102.
3. Ibid., p. 157.
4. Ibid., p. 207.
5. Ibid., p. 267.
6. Ibid., p. 295.

GROUP PRAYER REQUESTS   TODAY'S DATE:_____

NAME	REQUEST	RESULTS

EXTENDING GRACE

MEMORY VERSE
And whatever you do, whether in word or deed,
do it all in the name of the Lord Jesus, giving
thanks to God the Father through him.
Colossians 3:17

When you receive the grace God extends to you, your thoughts, attitudes and actions are transformed. As your heart grows closer to His and you become more like Jesus, you will learn to extend grace to others. Extending grace to others is vital to the Body of Christ and to your witness to the rest of the world. In this week's study we are going to explore different ways that you can extend grace to those around you.

DAY 1: *Serving*

Think about the myriad ways that the members of the Body of Christ can serve one another. We have all been gifted to serve one another. If you are unsure about what spiritual gifts you've been given, pray for God to reveal those gifts He has given you.[1]

>> According to Ephesians 1:22-23, who is the head of the Body—the Church? What is the significance of His position?

>> What does 1 Corinthians 12:12-27 tell us about our position in the Body of Christ?

➢ Read verses 15 and 16 again and think about them in relationship to your own body. Is there one part of your body that you would willingly give up? Why or why not?

When you became a member of the family of God, you immediately became a part of the Body of Christ. Just as there are different parts of the body, there are different spiritual gifts. It is important that you minister to one another according to the spiritual gifts you have been given by the Holy Spirit.

➢ What are the spiritual gifts listed in Romans 12:6-8?

➢ Thinking about some of the Christians you know, can you identify spiritual gifts that were not listed in Romans 12:6-8?

There are many, many spiritual gifts in the Body of Christ. One way to know if you are serving in your particular area of gifting is if you are experiencing a feeling of obligation, burden and stress instead of feeling fulfilled and peaceful knowing you are using your gifts to serve the Lord. This is not to say that when you identify and serve in your gifted area that you will not experience highs and lows while doing so. It does mean that when you are truly serving the Lord using the spiritual gifts He has given you, you will know it by the feelings of satisfaction you experience.

➢ How has someone ministered to you through his or her spiritual gifts?

What was this person's general attitude toward serving the Lord?

O God, by Your grace, I am what I am! Your grace has healed and overshadowed my sinful past [see 1 Corinthians 15:10].

Thank You that I am a part of Your Body. I ask that You would help me recognize and understand the gifts You've given so that I can effectively serve my brothers and sisters in Christ.

I pray that everything I do will be done with the strength You provide so that in all things You may be praised and receive all the glory! [see 1 Peter 4:11].

DAY 2: *Forgiving*

Forgiveness has been addressed several times in this study. There is a reason. Forgiveness—whether giving or receiving it—is one of the keys to freedom in Christ. If you are dealing with issues of unforgiveness, it will seriously affect your ability to experience God's freedom.

➤ Read Matthew 6:14. How have you experienced forgiveness—whether needing it or extending it—in a relationship?

What was the end result of this experience? Did it change the dynamics of your relationship with this person? In what way?

≫ Have you ever prayed for someone when you were truly angry with him or her?

❑ Yes ❑ No

If yes, place an *X* on the following scale to mark how angry you were when you first began to pray:

1	2	3	4	5
Irritated		Very Angry		Furious

Did your anger subside during your prayer time?

❑ Yes ❑ No

When you pray for someone, you are going before the Lord on that person's behalf. If you humble yourself and allow God to help you see that person through His eyes, your heart will begin to soften toward him or her. When your heart is softened, you cannot hold on to anger. It is only with a heart softened by God that you can extend His grace toward others.

O God, I praise You for Your unconditional love and forgiveness. I pray that I will quickly humble my heart when I need to seek or extend forgiveness.

Forgiving Lord, remind me and give me the strength to confess my sins to another in order that I may be healed and so that my prayers will not be hindered [see James 5:16].

DAY 3: *Listening and Validating*

We all have a desire to feel heard and validated. This is an essential element of any healthy relationship. Sometimes, however, listening to someone and validating that person take great patience and self-control. It can be hard to allow someone to vent without feeling the urge to jump into the fray with your own opinions on the situation.

✎ Read Proverbs 18:2,13 and James 1:19-20. How have you experienced this in your own life?

✎ What is the warning in James 1:26?

God has made it very clear: Careful *listening* before speaking is the best practice. When someone shares a heartache or disappointment, he or she is typically seeking validation, not a solution—so don't offer a solution unless you are asked! Simply listen with both ears, acknowledge the feelings being shared and attempt to understand where the other person is coming from. In this way, you validate and extend grace to that person.

✎ Why do you suppose the tongue is so hard to tame, as described in James 3:2-11?

How have you been hurt by another's untamed tongue? How have you hurt others?

✎ How has someone made you feel validated by carefully listening to you vent your feelings?

The most important way of validating another person is to listen carefully as he or she speaks. When someone is angry or upset, allow that person to express the emotions he or she is feeling without passing judgment or trying to solve the problem.

O God, in order to bring about the righteous life that You desire, I pray that I would be quick to listen and slow to speak. Help me to be thoughtful and understanding as I listen [see James 1:19].

Help me to listen before I answer. Help me to validate and extend grace whenever someone is sharing his or her thoughts or feelings with me [see Proverbs 18:13].

DAY 4: *Accepting*

Have you ever wondered how it is that Christians struggle with repeated sin? Have you ever sat in judgment of a fellow believer? After all, those who have not accepted Christ will continue to live sinful lives—that's a given, right? But someone who knows the truth and has given his or her life to Christ should know better. And shouldn't that Christian be held accountable for his or her behavior? Well, before you go pointing out the faults of others, consider what the Word has to say about judging and accepting others.

➤ According to 1 Corinthians 4:4-5, who alone can judge the motives of a person's heart?

➤ According to Matthew 7:1-5, when you are busy judging others, what happens to your focus?

When you stop monitoring your own words and actions, what can happen to your own walk with the Lord?

We all struggle with sin, even after becoming Christians. We are not called to judge one another but to accept one another with the love of Christ. It is important to note that acceptance of someone does not mean acceptance of his or her sinful behavior. Instead of standing in judgment of someone, the Word tells us to speak "the truth in love" (Ephesians 4:15). In fact, in Ephesians 4, which begins with the command to "live a life worthy of the calling you have received" (v. 1), we are reminded over and over that we are to remain unified in the Body of Christ.

➤ According to John 13:20, who are we ultimately accepting when we accept others?

When you look past the weaknesses of others and love and accept others with the love of Christ, your honor of them and your extension of grace to them directly affect your relationship with the One who has accepted you and extended grace to you in spite of your sin.

O God, I believe what Your Word says, that I will be judged in the same way that I judge others. Father, forgive me for looking at the specks in others' eyes and not paying attention to the planks in my own eyes. Help me to extend the same measure of grace You have given me [see Matthew 7:1-5].

Lord, bring to light the hidden sins and motives of my heart so that I would be blameless before You when You return. Teach me to accept others and leave the judging of their motives to You [see 1 Corinthians 4:5].

DAY 5: *Assuming*

Assuming you know what motivates another person can be fatal to any relationship. When we assume, we become judge and jury over another person. As we learned yesterday, God is the only One who knows the true motives in anyone's heart and He also knows the hurts, trials and difficulties with which he or she must live.

In Proverbs 16:2 we are told that we cannot judge a person's motive. The best way to arm yourself against the destructive nature of assuming is to communicate, ask questions and discuss issues before hurt feelings or anger occur.

➤ According to 2 Timothy 2:22-24, how can we avoid quarrels?

➤ How does Romans 12:18 relate to being careful not to assume the motives of others?

There will be times when the person you are asking questions of may not be completely candid in his or her response. Don't take this as a sign that he or she has something to hide. The person may just be reticent or even unsure of how to express him- or herself.

➤ Proverbs 16:28 pointedly refers to gossip. How does gossip adversely affect relationships?

Remember that only God knows what is in anyone's heart. If you have tried discussing a situation with someone and still feel that there is something amiss, talk to the Lord in prayer about the person and leave the situation with Him. Let God work out the details. Honor your relationship with that person by extending grace toward him or her—and most of all, "trust in the LORD with all your heart and lean not on your own understanding" (Proverbs 3:5).

 O God, help me to pursue righteousness, faith, love and peace, along with those who call on the Lord out of a pure heart; that I would be kind to everyone, able to teach, and guard my heart from resentment [see 2 Timothy 2:22-24].

Father, I pray that I would always believe the best about people, especially if I am unwilling to ask questions. Help me to seek out reconciliation whenever I am confused or feeling hurt by something that was said or done. I pray that I would honor and extend grace to every relationship You have so lovingly given me.

DAY 6: *Reflections*

In this week's study, we have explored different ways to extend grace to those in the Body of Christ and also how to be an example of that grace to unbelievers. In this fast-paced, busy world it is easy to get so caught up in the daily routines of life that serving others often gets placed on the back burner. Take your relationship with the Lord seriously, live completely devoted to and desperately dependent on Him, and become passionately Christ centered. When you do, you will have opportunity after opportunity to extend grace to others who desperately need it.

As you think about ways that you can extend grace to others, also take a look at how well and how often you extend grace to your family. Oftentimes they are the last to be recipients of your grace.

Equally important is extending grace to yourself. If you have not yet reached the goal you set for yourself at this point in your First Place journey, don't be discouraged. Would you extend grace and encouragement to someone else who had not yet reached his or her goals? Of course! Pick yourself up, dust yourself off, and keep moving toward your goals. God is with you every step of the way.

Merciful God, thank You for opening my eyes and turning them from darkness to light, and from the power of Satan to God, so that I may receive forgiveness of sins and a place among those who are sanctified by faith in You [see Acts 26:18].[2]

Father, Your Word teaches that You humble and test Your children so that in the end it might go well with them. You do not humble and test us to bring us low and cause us to fail but to teach us how to succeed in You [see Deuteronomy 8:16].[3]

Father God, I ask You to lead me when I'm blinded by ways I have not known, along unfamiliar paths. Please guide me, Lord, turn the darkness into light before me and make the rough places smooth. I know You will not forsake me [see Isaiah 42:16].[4]

DAY 7: *Reflections*

We have studied the *how-to* of extending grace this week, but before we move on, let's look at the *why*. This week's memory verse articulates it perfectly: "Whatever you do . . . do it all in the name of the Lord Jesus." It's all for Him, for His glory and praise.

When we extend grace to others, it can be easy to give in to pride, feeling that we've done some great thing. Serving, forgiving, listening, accepting and not assuming are noteworthy, but we must not forget who gives us the strength to do these things. Without the power of the Holy Spirit, we would fall flat on our face every time!

As the Holy Spirit empowers you to live righteously in freedom, don't forget to give glory to whom it is due. Check your heart often, making sure it is clothed in humility. And don't be shy in proclaiming the transforming power of the Holy Spirit! Both unbelievers and believers alike will benefit when you give Jesus Christ all the credit for the grace you extend them.

God, according to Your steadfast Word, pride only breeds quarrels, but wisdom is found in those who take advice. My pride has caused such conflict, Lord! Please help me to humble myself and receive Your wisdom [see Proverbs 13:10].[5]

Lord, please help me not miss the grace of God. Help me see that no bitter root grows up in me to cause trouble and defile many [see Hebrews 12:15].[6]

If I do not judge, I will not be judged. If I do not condemn, I will not be condemned. If I forgive, I will be forgiven. Help me, Lord, to extend more grace so that I will continue to receive more grace [see Luke 6:37].[7]

Notes

1. For more information on spiritual gifts, see C. Peter Wagner, *Discovering Your Spiritual Gifts* (Ventura, CA: Regal Books, 2002).

2. Beth Moore, *Praying God's Word* (Nashville, TN: Broadman and Holman, 2000), p. 47.

3. Ibid., p. 63.

4. Ibid., p. 115.

5. Ibid., p. 131.

6. Ibid., p. 157.

7. Ibid., p. 225.

GROUP PRAYER REQUESTS   TODAY'S DATE:_____

NAME	REQUEST	RESULTS

IMPARTING GRACE

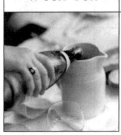

MEMORY VERSE

Therefore go and make disciples of all nations, . . . teaching them to obey everything I have commanded you. And surely I am with you always, to the very end of the age.

Matthew 28:19-20

Imparting grace is simply showing and telling others about God's grace. God not only calls us to extend grace to others, but He also calls us to introduce others to His grace and transforming power; He calls us to make disciples. Making disciples may sound intimidating; you may feel like you are barely getting the hang of things yourself! But remember the final declaration of the verse: "Surely I am with you always, to the very end of the age." Ask the Lord this week to drive out any fear hiding in your heart as we explore the process of imparting grace.

DAY 1: *Being*

As Christians, we are called to share Christ with others, not just in words and deeds but also through who we *are* and how we live. Our faith, our love of God, must not be merely skin deep; we must embrace our relationship with Jesus with our soul and allow it to permeate every area of our life. We must first *be* His disciple before we can make disciples.

➺ Think about someone you know who not only appears to live a godly life but also consistently exhibits authentic Christian life. What is it about this person that enables you to see that his or her love for the Lord is not just for show?

Are you inspired by this person? Does he or she make you want to walk even closer to the Lord? How does this person inspire nonbelievers and believers with his or her life?

≫ Read Titus 2, in which Paul explained what a godly life must exhibit and how to model Christ to others. List the attributes we must be teaching and showing to others.

It is important to ask yourself, *Is my personal and private life consistent with the way I talk and act around other Christians?* Are you a Sunday-only believer who is on your best behavior at church or in public, appearing on the outside to be a good Christian? Or are you a full-time believer whose faith is reflected not only at church and in public but also at home when you're relaxing with your family and friends? Remember, in order to share the good news of Jesus Christ with others, you must make sure that your own life reflects the grace He has given you.

 O Mighty God, I ask that You would empower me by Your Holy Spirit to *be* the person You have called me to be according to Your Word and Your model, Jesus Christ.

Father, help me live according to Your Spirit both in public and in private. May my mind dwell on what the Spirit desires every minute of the day, so I may enjoy the benefits of life and peace [see Romans 8:5-6].

DAY 2: *Mentoring*

Mentoring is a ministry of grace and reconciliation. Mentoring means helping others understand and experience the joy that comes from having an intimate relationship with God. It requires an investment of time and energy in the life of another person. For those called to minister His grace through mentoring, 2 Corinthians 5:17-21 paints the perfect picture.

➤ After God reconciled us to Himself, what did He give to us (v. 18)?

What has He committed to us (v. 19)?

➤ In Titus 2, Paul referred to older men and women teaching—or mentoring—younger ones (vv. 2-3). Does this mean you cannot mentor someone who is older than you? Why or why not?

You may be mature in your faith because you accepted Christ long ago and have continued to grow in your relationship with Him. This makes you an older, or more mature, Christian than someone perhaps older than you chronologically who has just recently accepted Christ. You can successfully mentor that person in learning about God as he or she begins to follow the Lord.

➤ Name at least one person who has been a mentor to you. How has that person helped you to grow and mature as a Christian?

Just as you mentor others, it is also important that you have a mentor who can encourage you as you continue to mature in your faith. If you don't already have a mentor or someone to mentor, pray that God would bring the right person into your life for that purpose.

O Father God, I bow before You with a humble heart, understanding that You have reconciled my evil heart to Yours. Thank You for Your grace.

Gracious Lord, You have administered to me the ministry of reconciliation. Empower me by Your Spirit to be Christ's ambassador as though You were making Your appeal through me; that as I am reconciled to You, Father, I would minister Your reconciliation to other believers [see 2 Corinthians 5:18-20].

DAY 3: *Teaching*

As you mature in Christ, you may find that one of the gifts God has given you is the ability to teach others. Historically, many Christians have taught in formal and informal settings—it has been a rite of passage that symbolized spiritual knowledge and maturity. For this and other reasons, many of us are intimidated by the thought of teaching others in a Bible study, small group (such as a First Place meeting) or other setting.

This hesitation is not completely unfounded. The Bible is clear that teaching others carries with it a great responsibility.

➤ What warning is found in James 3:1?

Why would James give such a warning?

➤ Who has been an influential teacher in your life? Describe how this person has inspired you.

Teaching puts you in a position in which the eyes of others are focused on you. It also gives you the potential to be very influential in the lives of others. For these reasons it is essential that you have a firm foundation of faith and biblical knowledge before you begin to teach others.

Take to heart Paul's admonition to Timothy in 2 Timothy 3:16-17. The work and discipline that go into teaching others will be in vain if you don't know what you are talking about! It's imperative that you study the Word yourself before you attempt to teach others.

Now so far, this has all been pretty discouraging, hasn't it? Who would want to teach if it requires so much work, only to be judged by a higher standard? God sets the bar high (for obvious reasons), but He also greatly blesses those who teach. There is incredible satisfaction in leading others to the wellspring of God's grace—and it can lead you to examine your own heart daily, bringing you to greater intimacy with the Lord. The benefits far outweigh the costs!

Teaching can take many forms—the subjects and settings are limitless. However, there are some essentials.

➣ What things are women to teach, according to Titus 2:4-5?

➣ What are men to teach (vv. 6-8)?

These verses highlight things that every believer should be teaching others, at least informally. Parents have the responsibility to teach their own children as well (see Deuteronomy 6:4-9). If you feel that God has given you the spiritual gift of teaching, and you are ready spiritually, find a mentor who teaches others—someone with knowledge and preparation and organization skills who is willing to share his or her insights with you. Attend a class he or she is currently teaching and take notes. Ask about techniques and materials that have worked. Ask the teacher to share some of the struggles he or she had when first beginning to teach, including fears, failures and humorous accounts. Through all of this, you will be able to see the human side of teaching, and as a result, it may not seem so intimidating.

Lord, I know that You have appointed Your children to minister to others in many different ways. My heart is open to following your direction—even to teach—so that the Body of Christ may be built up and become mature, attaining to the whole measure of the fullness of Christ [see Ephesians 4:11-13].

Father God, You have appointed me to bear fruit—fruit that will last. As I mature and develop a more intimate relationship with You, dispel any fear in my heart that might keep me from teaching others [see John 15:16].

DAY 4: *Entrusting*

Last week's Scripture memory verse, Colossians 3:17, reminded us of our motive in extending grace: "Do it all in the name of the Lord Jesus." The same is true in imparting grace. Unless we remember that our sole purpose is to bring God glory and that apart from Him we can do nothing, our pride will sabotage our efforts.

From the moment we begin to lead someone, we must entrust that person to God, relying on His strength and wisdom. We have to give up any claim we think we might have on the other person or his or her growth and remember that any good that results from our instruction is solely the result of God's intervention and grace. We can take none of the credit, nor can we bear the burden of thinking that another's sanctification depends on us.

➤ According to Philippians 1:6, who begins the process of salvation and sanctification?

Who completes it?

Understanding that principle relieves a lot of pressure, doesn't it? No matter how gifted you are in imparting grace to others, you will watch brothers and sisters stumble—and even fall away. You cannot control another's will—even God chooses not to control our wills. Satan will try to use difficult situations to discourage you from teaching and mentoring others. But don't give in to his guilt. Remember that God ultimately begins and finishes the work in each of our lives.

>> Have you ever watched a friend make poor choices, or even fall away from the faith? How did it affect you?

Part of entrusting someone to God is remembering that He may have to take that person through deep valleys and dark nights in order to finish the work He started in him or her. Don't ever give up hope; that person is in better hands than you could ever offer!

Perhaps the most important aspect of entrusting is prayer. According to James 5:16, "The prayer of a righteous man is powerful and effective." Commit yourself to pray for those whom God has put in your life. As you pray for their spiritual walk and intimacy with God, you will not only be encouraged, but you will also protect your heart from swelling up with pride. Pray for their specific needs—that God would give you the words they need to hear and that your actions would match your words.

Father, I know that imparting grace to others is a huge responsibility—one that I can't handle on my own. Thank You that You will complete every good work You begin, whether or not I am the perfect mentor [see Philippians 1:6].

O Lord, You are able to do immeasurably more than all we ask or imagine, and it is Your power that is at work within us. To You be all glory throughout all generations, for ever and ever! Amen [see Ephesians 3:20-21].

DAY 5: *Harvesting*

When you impart grace to others, a harvest naturally follows. The harvest season may not come when you think it should—and you may never see the results of your efforts—but God has a divine green thumb. He can help anyone grow. All He asks is that we attend to the tasks He has given us.

➤ In 1 Corinthians 3:5-7, what task did God give Paul?

What task was given to Apollo?

What was the result of their service?

When we are obedient to the Lord by attending to the tasks He has given us, we also reap a harvest of blessing for ourselves. Do you realize how often you are rewarded for your faithfulness and obedience to the Lord?

➤ Identify ways God has rewarded you in the past for your obedience.

➤ According to 1 Corinthians 9:24-25, how long does your reward last?

We're all in this freedom race together. As we fight for our freedom every day, we can fight for the freedom of others as well. As we minister grace to others, the enemy hates it and will fight back. However, greater is He who is in us than he who is in the world (see 1 John 4:4). We have already overcome as we run the race. Like Paul, we will receive a crown that will last forever (see 1 Corinthians 9:25).

≫ In 1 Thessalonians 2:17-20, Paul was writing of his longing to see the church in Thessalonica. What was his hope?

Those whom you minister to and mentor are a crown to you—not so that you can boast; rather, so that you can glory in the Lord, laying your crown at His feet, committing those in your care back to Him, the One who will change their lives.

Living by example, mentoring, teaching and entrusting can be downright exhausting! But the harvest, including receiving God's blessings for your obedience and watching others grow in Christ, makes every minute of sacrifice worthwhile.

O God, empower me by Your Spirit to run the race that I would run in such a way as to win the crown that will last forever [see 1 Corinthians 9:24-25].

I thank You that those to whom You minister through me are a hope and joy to me, and the crown in which I will glory in You [see 1 Thessalonians 2:19].

Father, help me to persevere under trials and tests that come with imparting grace to others. For then I will receive the crown of life that You have promised to those who love You [see James 1:12].

DAY 6: *Reflections*

In this week's study, you have gained insight into what it means to "make disciples." It is a natural outpouring of the supernatural work of the Holy Spirit in your life. Although living an honorable and reverent life is not easy, nor without battles from time to time, sharing the grace of Jesus with others is an automatic response when He indwells your heart and life. Being a disciple, mentoring, teaching, entrusting and harvesting are privileges beyond anything the world can offer. Consider Jack's story:

> Jack was thrust into the biggest trial of his life when his wife walked out on him. Almost immediately the Lord placed an older godly man in his life. This man was available day and night. An important key to Jack's healing during this time was that every time he wanted to give up and lose hope, his mentor would direct him to God's Word. They would always look at what God's Word said about his situation that day. They literally took one day at a time. Jack learned to pray the Word, and as he did so, God's peace and joy came back into his life and the healing began. Instead of becoming dependent on his mentor for peace and comfort, he learned to depend on God's Word and His Spirit. As a result, God displayed His faithfulness and over time Jack's wife yielded her heart to the Lord. God gave them a new life, blessed by Him.

God, in His faithfulness, placed that mentor in Jack's life at his weakest moments. When Jack was weary, disillusioned and confused, God displayed His strength and brought guidance and support to Jack when he needed it most. Only God knows what would have happened had that mentor not made the commitment to follow God's call by imparting grace to Jack.

Lord God, teach me knowledge and good judgment, for I believe in Your commands [see Psalm 119:66].[1]

O Lord, I want You to say of me, "I know your deeds, your love and faith, your service and perseverance, and that you are now doing more than you did at first" [Revelation 2:19]. Cause these words to be true of my life, Father.[2]

Like the apostle Paul, help me serve You, Lord, with great humility and with tears, even when I am severely tested [see Acts 20:19].[3]

DAY 7: *Reflections*

Over and over we have seen that God's grace encompasses every aspect of life. There is not an area in each of our lives that God does not take interest in or doesn't care about. As you have worked on the Nine Commitments, God has been at work in and for you. He has empowered you to tread forward in the battle for your freedom and live out the victory He has already won for you. As you submit to Him and desperately depend on Him, allow him total and complete access to your heart. He loves you so much and has given you everything you need to experience His grace and the abundant life He has prepared for you. Believe His Word and receive His peace, His joy, His hope and His love.

Beloved, don't allow the enemy to steal these promises or accomplishments from you. Stand firm in that which you know to be true. God's Word is true. Continue studying, praying, confessing and believing His Word in the face of difficulty. Don't allow a day to go by without confessing your sins and your need for Him. Only then can you experience victory, peace and joy, which is beautifully and lovingly packaged in His grace.

 I thank You, my God, who always leads me in triumphal procession in Christ and through me desires to spread everywhere the fragrance of the knowledge of Him. For You have called me to be the aroma of Christ among those who are being saved and those who are perishing [see 2 Corinthians 2:14-15].[4]

Father, Your Word says that he who walks with the wise grows wise, but a companion of fools suffers harm. Please surround me with the right kind of companions [see Proverbs 13:20].[5]

Lord God, cause my work to be produced by faith, my labor prompted by love, and my endurance inspired by hope in my Lord Jesus Christ [see 1 Thessalonians 1:3].[6]

Notes
1. Beth Moore, *Praying God's Word* (Nashville, TN: Broadman and Holman, 2000), p. 39.
2. Ibid., p. 55.
3. Ibid., p. 68.
4. Ibid., p. 114.
5. Ibid., p. 132.
6. Ibid., p. 266

GROUP PRAYER REQUESTS   TODAY'S DATE:_____

NAME	REQUEST	RESULTS

FOOD EXCHANGES MADE EASY

Don't let the phrase "food exchanges" intimidate you—although it may sound very technical, it really is just a simple method of measuring calorie and nutrient values of foods. Dietitians have used food exchanges for years to help others maintain healthy eating habits, and you can use them to create a well-balanced diet for yourself.

There are seven food-exchange groups: meat, bread/starch, vegetable, fruit, milk, fat and free foods. The First Place Live-It plan gives you a variety of foods from which to choose in each of the seven groups so that you can plan tasty meals without boring repetition of the same foods over and over again. Remember: Foods from *all* groups are necessary to good health—no one group supplies everything you need for a well-balanced, healthy diet.

The wellness worksheets for this study are interactive and will aid you in learning how to accurately determine exchanges for each of the seven food-exchange groups. (For more information on the answers to the quiz questions, refer to pages 45-64 in your *First Place Member's Guide.*)

HELPFUL TIPS

- Exchanges are usually expressed as ounces or standard measuring cups and spoons. As you are learning about figuring exchanges, you will want to weigh and measure your food choices. You'll need a small dietary scale for weighing meat. As you become more familiar with the measurements, you'll be able to recognize quantities (e.g., ½ cup peas or 1 cup puffed cereal).
- Work to memorize the calorie limit for each food exchange (e.g., 1 bread/starch exchange contains 80 calories). This will help you determine exchanges for foods not listed in the Live-It plan. For example, let's say a box of crackers has 40 calories per 1-ounce serving. Using the equation "How many exchanges equal 40 calories," you would know that 1 serving of crackers equals ½ bread/starch exchange. Likewise, 2 servings of the crackers (2 ounces) would give you 1 bread/starch exchange. Knowing the calorie limits for each

food-exchange group is important to making food choices on items not listed specifically in the Live-It Food Plan section of the *First Place Member's Guide.*

Meat Exchanges

All foods in the meat exchange list provide generous amounts of protein, the nutrient responsible for tissue building and repair. These foods also contain similar amounts of all nutrients, except fat. Meat exchanges are divided into three groups according to their fat content—choose foods from the lean-meat section as often as you can (and avoid fried meats). With the exception of peanut butter and fish, the fat found in meat choices is saturated fat, which should be avoided as much as possible according to health officials.

🍎 1 ounce lean meat contains _____ calories, _____ grams of protein and _____ grams of fat.

🍎 1 ounce medium-fat meat contains _____ calories, _____ grams of protein and _____ grams of fat.

🍎 1 ounce high-fat meat contains _____ calories, _____ grams of protein and _____ grams of fat.

🍎 1 ounce lean meat equals _____ meat exchange(s).

🍎 1 ounce medium-fat meat equals _____ meat exchange(s) plus _____ fat exchange(s).

🍎 1 ounce high-fat meat equals _____ meat exchange(s) plus _____ fat exchange(s).

It is important to weigh or measure meat servings. Exchanges are based on the weight of the meat after cooking. (For example, 4 ounces of uncooked meat will usually weigh about 3 ounces when cooked.)

- 3 ounces top round steak equal _____ meat exchange(s).

- _____ cup(s) tuna, packed in water, equal(s) 1 meat exchange.

- _____ egg whites equal(s) 1 meat exchange.

- 1 egg equals _____ meat exchange(s) plus _____ fat exchange(s).

- 3 ounces chicken with skin equal _____ meat exchange(s) plus _____ fat exchange(s).

- Medium-fat cheese will have _____ grams of fat per ounce.

- 2 ounces ribs equal _____ meat exchange(s) plus _____ fat exchange(s).

- 1 tablespoon peanut butter equals _____ meat exchange(s) plus _____ fat exchange(s).

Answers: 55, 7, 3, 75, 7, 5, 100, 7, 8, 1, 1, ½, 1, 1, 3, ¼, 3, 1, ½, 3, 1½, 5, 2, 2, 1, 1

BREAD/STARCH EXCHANGES

Bread/starch exchanges are your daily energy supplies. Together with vegetable and fruit exchanges, these furnish carbohydrates—your body's primary fuels—which are necessary to burn fat efficiently. Choosing whole-grain products is very important as you make bread/starch exchange choices.

🍎 Each bread/starch exchange contains _____ calories.

🍎 This includes _____ carbohydrates (in grams), _____ proteins (in grams) and _____ fats (in grams).

🍎 _____ slice(s) of white or whole-wheat bread equal(s) 1 bread/starch exchange.

🍎 _____ cup(s) cooked cereal equal(s) 1 bread/starch exchange.

🍎 _____ cracker(s) equal(s) 1 bread/starch exchange.

Except for prepared bread/starch exchanges, there is almost no fat in the bread/starch exchange group. It is very important to watch for hidden _____ in this group when choosing processed foods. The more processed a food is, the more each serving size should be decreased and the fat content should be increased. For example:

🍎 _____ ounce(s) baked potato equal(s) 1 bread/starch exchange

🍎 _____ ounce(s) French fries equal(s) 1 bread/starch exchange plus 1 fat exchange.

🍎 _____ ounce(s) potato chips equal(s) 1 bread/starch exchange plus 2 fat exchanges.

Serving sizes not only get smaller with each processing step, but valuable nutrients are also lost.

Be aware that some bread/starch exchanges contain fats. One gram of fat per serving is not counted, but if a food choice has 2 to 3 grams of fat, add _____ fat exchange(s). If a food choice has 4 to 5 grams of fat, add 1 fat exchange. For example:

🍎 1 6-inch flour tortilla equals _____ bread/starch exchange(s) plus _____ fat exchange(s).

🍎 1 2-inch biscuit equals _____ bread/starch exchange(s) plus _____ fat exchange(s).

🍎 1 2- to 4-inch pancake equals _____ bread/starch exchange(s) plus _____ fat exchange(s).

Fiber is extremely important to good health. Aim for 25 to 35 grams or more of fiber each day. Carefully choose products listed as whole-grain products.

Answers: 80, 15, 3, trace, 1, $\frac{1}{2}$, 6, fats, 3, 1$\frac{1}{2}$, 1, $\frac{1}{2}$, 1, $\frac{1}{2}$, 1, 1, 1, 2

VEGETABLE EXCHANGES

Vegetables supply valuable vitamins and minerals. Scientific research has proven that vegetables actually aid in preventing major diseases. A key to choosing vegetables is to think in terms of color: Vegetables that are bright or dark in color usually provide more nutrients. The generous use of an assortment of nutritious vegetables in your diet contributes to sound health and vitality, so enjoy ample amounts of cooked and raw vegetables.

- Each vegetable exchange has _____ calories.

- Each vegetable exchange has _____ carbohydrates (in grams), _____ proteins (in grams) and _____ fat (in grams).

- A minimum of _____ servings from the vegetable exchange is suggested.

- _____ to _____ vegetable exchanges per day are encouraged.

- Avoid _____ vegetables.

- Any fat added during preparation must be counted as a _____.

- A serving of vegetables usually contains _____ to _____ grams of _____.

- Vegetables are naturally low in _____ and _____.

- Salads should contain _____ amounts of lettuce and large amounts of other vegetables high in nutrients.

The vegetables listed on the free vegetable list have fewer than 25 calories per 1-cup serving. The maximum raw serving amount for each to count as a free vegetable is as follows:

VEGETABLE	SERVING SIZE
Alfalfa sprouts	2 cups
Cabbage	1 cup
Celery	1 cup
Chinese cabbage	2 cups
Cress, garden	1 cup
Cucumber	2 cups
Endive	3 cups
Green onion	2 cups
Lettuce	3 cups
Mushrooms	1 cup sliced
Radishes	1 cup
Romaine lettuce	2 cups
Spinach	2 cups
Watercress	6 cups
Zucchini	1 cup

Answers: 25, 5, 2, 0, 2, 3, 4, frying, fat exchange, 2, 3, fiber, fat, sodium, small

FRUIT EXCHANGES

Fruits are full of energy-producing carbohydrates and are a valuable source of vitamins, minerals and fiber. Sweet by nature, most fruits do not need additional sweetening and can be used as a refreshing addition to a meal or as a satisfying snack.

It is important to read labels carefully to determine if sugar has been added to canned, frozen or dried fruit. Many juices and syrup-packed fruit will add unwanted calories.

🍎 Each fruit exchange has _____ calories and _____ carbohydrates.

🍎 Most fruits have _____ grams of fiber.

🍎 _____ fruit, such as grapes, can be a great snack.

🍎 _____ bananas, strawberries and other fruits allows them to be saved for great First Place smoothies or milkshakes.

🍎 _____ cup(s) unsweetened applesauce equal(s) 1 fruit exchange.

🍎 _____ of a 9-inch banana (_____ ounces) equals 1 fruit exchange.

🍎 _____ of a cantaloupe (_____ ounces) or _____ cup(s) cubed cantaloupe equals 1 fruit exchange.

🍎 _____ small grapes equal 1 fruit exchange.

🍎 _____ ring(s) or _____ ounce(s) dried apples equal(s) 1 fruit exchange.

_____ tablespoons (_____ ounce) raisins equal one fruit exchange.

It is important to learn the serving sizes of fruits. Keep in mind that if you have a need or desire for extra exchanges, the fruit exchange list is the *second* best from which to choose; the vegetable exchange list should be your first choice.

Answers: 60, 15, 2, Frozen, Freezing, $\frac{1}{2}$, $\frac{1}{2}$, 3, $\frac{1}{3}$, 7, 1, 17, 4, $\frac{3}{4}$, 2, $\frac{3}{4}$

148   *Living in Grace*

MILK EXCHANGES

Milk products (including yogurt) are the leading source of dietary calcium. The milk exchange list is divided into sections according to fat content. While up to 3 grams of fat are allowed for a lean meat exchange, this is not true for milk exchanges. For example: One serving of cheese containing 3 grams of fat is considered lean meat. However, if that cheese were to be counted as a milk exchange, the 3 grams of fat would also be counted as a fat exchange.

- 1 cup nonfat milk contains _____ calories, _____ carbohydrates (in grams), _____ protein (in grams) and _____ fat (in grams).

- 1 cup 1% milk contains _____ calories, _____ carbohydrates (in grams), _____ protein (in grams) and _____ fat (in grams).

- 1 cup 2% milk contains _____ calories, _____ carbohydrates (in grams), _____ protein (in grams) and _____ fat(s) (in grams).

- 1 cup whole milk contains _____ calories, _____ carbohydrates (in grams), _____ protein (in grams) and _____ fat(s) (in grams).

- 1 cup nonfat milk equals _____ milk exchange(s).

- 1 cup 1% milk equals _____ milk exchange(s) and _____ fat exchange(s).

- 1 cup 1½ % or 2% milk equals _____ milk exchange(s) and _____ fat exchange(s).

- 1 cup whole milk equals _____ milk exchange(s) and _____ fat exchange(s).

🍎 _____ cup(s) dry nonfat milk equal(s) 1 milk exchange.

🍎 8 ounces fat-free, artificially sweetened dairy yogurt equal _____ milk exchange(s).

🍎 8 ounces low-fat, sugar-free dairy yogurt equal _____ milk exchange(s) and _____ fat exchange(s).

🍎 Pudding (sugar-free) prepared with fat-free milk equals _____ milk exchange(s) and _____ bread/starch exchange(s).

FAT EXCHANGES

Not only do fats provide energy and ward off hunger sensations, but they are also vital for transporting minerals and vitamins throughout your body. Although necessary to a healthy diet, fats can pack a lot of calories in deceptively small parcels and are often hidden in foods. Health officials advise us to stay away from saturated fats and trans fats as much as possible and to choose unsaturated fats instead. It is very important to our physical well-being to consume healthy choices from the fat exchange list each day, but be very careful to stay within daily fat recommendations.

- Each fat exchange contains _____ calories and _____ grams of fat.

- 1 gram of fat contains _____ calories, while 1 gram of protein or 1 gram of carbohydrate contains only 4 calories.

- Saturated fat is found in _____ and _____ ___ products.

- _____ avocado equals 1 fat exchange.

- _____ teaspoon(s) margarine equal(s) 1 fat exchange.

- _____ tablespoon(s) diet margarine equal(s) 1 fat exchange.

- _____ teaspoon(s) mayonnaise equal(s) 1 fat exchange.

- _____ tablespoon(s) light mayonnaise equal(s) 1 fat exchange.

- _____ teaspoon(s) peanut butter equal(s) 1 fat exchange.[1]

- _____ tablespoon(s) chopped nuts equal(s) 1 fat exchange.

🍎 _____ peanuts or _____ pecans equal 1 fat exchange.

🍎 _____ teaspoon(s) of any kind of oil equal(s) 1 fat exchange.

Be sure and read salad-dressing labels carefully to find the number of fat grams per serving. There are some fat-free salad dressings that are high in calories, yet have zero fat grams. These do not count as a fat exchange and are considered a free food.

Answers: 45, 5, 9, animal, dairy, $\frac{1}{8}$, 1, 1, 1, 1, 1, 1, 10, 20, 1

Note

1. On the *Live-It Food Plan Video*, Molly Gee states that 2 teaspoons of peanut butter equal 1 fat exchange. The exact amount is 1 $\frac{1}{2}$ teaspoons. Molly Gee rounded the amount up to an even number of 2 teaspoons, and the Live-It plan has now rounded that figure down to an even amount of 1 teaspoon. You may choose the amount you feel is right for you.

FREE FOODS

The items listed on the Free Foods list are foods that do not have nutritional value and are usually very low in calories. First Place suggests that you try to keep these items below a total of _____ calories per day.

"Moderation" is a keyword used in all of First Place. Many items in the Free Foods list contain artificial sweeteners, so choosing too many could put you over the top of the "moderation theory." Choose wisely.

_____ free foods because all calories add up.

All _____ dressings are on this list. Be sure to check the calories; some are very high.

"Sugar-free" does not mean _____ free. Learn to check labels.

WATER

First Place recommends drinking _____ 8-ounce glasses of water each day.

Drinking eight 8-ounce glasses of water is good for your overall health and can aid in your weight loss. The best choice to meet this water requirement is to drink water; however, if you will not or cannot consume the eight glasses of water, then go to the next best thing. Your body will receive the benefits of water from any liquid you drink and from many of the foods that you choose. Choose the water you consume carefully—any liquids that contain artificial sweetener should be consumed in moderation. Many members find that using a straw or adding a lemon or an orange slice makes the water more palpable. If drinking eight glasses of water is difficult for you, begin with four and gradually increase the amount each day. If you were not drinking any water in the past, drinking two glasses each day is a great improvement. Celebrate the victory!

SUGAR

The amount of sugar that each First Place member chooses to eat is a personal choice. First Place does not have an exchange list for sugar. When you choose to eat a piece of candy, pie, cake, etc., write it on your CR and continue to eat your food-exchange allowance for that day. First Place encourages you to eat all your good food choices, such as fruits and vegetables, rather than exchange them for candy that has no nutritional value.

Answers: 50, Measure, fat-free, calorie, 8

FIRST PLACE
MENU PLANS

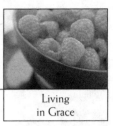

Each plan is based on approximately 1,400 calories.

Breakfast	0-1 meats, 1-2 breads, 1 fruit, 0-1 milk, 0-½ fat
Lunch	2 meats, 2 breads, 1 vegetable, 1 fruit, 1 fat
Dinner	3 meats, 2 breads, 2 vegetables, 1 fat
Snacks	1 bread, 1 fruit, 1 milk, ½-1 fat (or any remaining exchanges)

For more calories, add the following to the 1,400-calorie plan:

1,600 calories	2 breads, 1 fat
1,800 calories	2 meats, 3 breads, 1 vegetable, 1 fat
2,000 calories	2 meats, 4 breads, 1 vegetable, 3 fats
2,200 calories	2 meats, 5 breads, 1 vegetable, 1 fruit, 5 fats
2,400 calories	2 meats, 6 breads, 2 vegetables, 1 fruit, 6 fats

The exchanges for these meals were calculated using the MasterCook software. It uses a database of over 6,000 food items prepared using United States Department of Agriculture (USDA) publications and information from food manufacturers. As with any nutritional program, MasterCook calculates the nutritional values of the recipes based on ingredients. Nutrition may vary due to how the food is prepared, where the food comes from, soil content, season, ripeners, processing and methods of preparation. For these reasons, please use the recipes and menu plans as approximate guides. As always, consult your physician and/or a registered dietitian before starting a diet program.

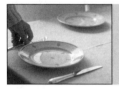

Note: We've included bonus recipes in this study's menu plans. Recipes for *italicized* items in menus can be found after each mealtime section.

🍎 Breakfast

⅓ medium cantaloupe or honeydew melon, topped with

1 c. artificially sweetened pineapple-flavored nonfat yogurt and

¼ c. Grape Nuts cereal

Exchanges: 1 ½ breads, 1 fruit, 1 milk

~~~~~~

1 c. puffed-rice cereal

½ medium banana

1 c. nonfat milk

Exchanges: 1 bread, 1 fruit, 1 milk

~~~~~~

Turkey Bacon, Potato and Egg Scramble

1 small banana

1 6-oz. container artificially sweetened nonfat yogurt (any flavor)

Exchanges: 1 meat, 1 bread, 1 fruit, 1 milk, ½ fat

~~~~~~

2 slices reduced-calorie sourdough toast

1 tsp. reduced-calorie margarine

¾ c. blueberries

1 c. nonfat milk

Exchanges: 2 breads, 1 fruit, 1 milk, ½ fat

~~~~~~

Cinnamon-Raisin French Toast

½ c. fresh fruit

1 c. nonfat milk

Exchanges: ½ meat, 2 breads, 1 fruit, 1 milk, ½ fat (Omit fat exchange if egg substitute is used.)

Raspberry-Banana Smoothie
1   slice whole-wheat toast, topped with
1   slice Kraft 2% milk sharp cheddar cheese
Exchanges: ½ meat, 1 bread, 2 fruits, 1 milk, ½ fat

~~~~~~

2   low-fat Eggo frozen waffles
½   c. unsweetened applesauce, mixed with
1   packet Splenda sugar substitute
½   c. raspberries
1   c. nonfat milk
Exchanges: 2 breads, ½ fruit, 1 milk, ½ fat

~~~~~~

1   c. prepared grits, mixed with
1   slice Kraft 2% sharp cheddar cheese, diced
½   c. nonfat milk
1   small banana
Exchanges: ½ meat, 2 breads, 1 fruit, ½ milk, ½ fat

~~~~~~

1 ½   c. Special K cereal
1   c. nonfat milk
1   c. sliced strawberries
Exchanges: 2 breads, 1 fruit, 1 milk

~~~~~~

1   packet instant Cream of Wheat
1   slice whole-wheat toast
1   tsp. reduced-calorie margarine
1   c. nonfat milk
Exchanges: 2 breads, 1 fruit, 1 milk, ½ fat

~~~~~~

1   packet Quaker Extra instant oatmeal
1   slice whole-wheat toast
½   medium banana
1   tsp. peanut butter
1   c. nonfat milk
Exchanges: 2 breads, 1 fruit, 1 milk, ½ fat

~~~~~~

Biscuits with Sausage Gravy

¾ c. orange juice

Exchanges: ½ meat, 2 breads, 1 fruit, ½ milk, 1 fat

~~~~~~

1 egg, poached or cooked with butter-flavored nonstick cooking spray

2 slices diet whole-wheat toast

1 small apple

1 c. nonfat milk

Exchanges: 1 meat, 1 bread, 1 fruit, 1 milk, ½ fat

~~~~~~

McDonald's Egg McMuffin

½ small banana

Exchanges: 2 meats, 2 breads, ½ fruit, 1 fat (Note: This is a high-meat and high-fat breakfast—adjust your menu plan accordingly.)

BONUS BREAKFAST RECIPES

Baked Grapefruit with Canadian Bacon and Muffin Sandwich

½ medium grapefruit

1 tsp. brown sugar

1 whole-wheat English muffin, split

1 oz. slice Canadian bacon

1 tomato slice

½ tsp. brown mustard

½ c. artificially sweetened vanilla-flavored nonfat yogurt

Preheat oven to 400° F. Place grapefruit skin-side down on nonstick cooking sheet and top with brown sugar. Bake 6 to 8 minutes; remove from oven (but don't remove grapefruit from cooking sheet). Arrange muffin halves on cooking sheet and top one half with bacon and other half with tomato. Return sheet to oven for 3 to 4 minutes. Remove from oven; spread mustard over bacon-topped muffin and together with other muffin half, create sandwich. Place grapefruit in bowl; top with yogurt and enjoy! Serves 1.

Exchanges: 1 meat, 2 breads, 1 fruit, ½ milk

~ ~

Biscuits with Sausage Gravy

6   oz. bulk turkey sausage
1   7½-oz. can (10 ct.) reduced-fat buttermilk biscuits
2   c. nonfat milk
2   tbsp. all-purpose flour
2   tsp. butter-flavored flakes (such as Molly McButter)
¼   tsp. black pepper
    Nonstick cooking spray

Preheat oven to 450° F. Arrange biscuits on nonstick baking sheet and set aside. Heat skillet coated with cooking spray over medium heat; crumble sausage into skillet and cook until thoroughly done. Drain any visible fat; return to skillet. When sausage is nearly done, combine milk, flour, butter-flavored flakes and pepper in medium bowl; mix well and add to skillet with sausage. Cook 8 minutes or until thickened, stirring occasionally with spatula to prevent sticking.

While gravy is cooking, place biscuits in oven; bake 5 to 6 minutes or until done. Split biscuits and arrange 4 halves on each serving plate; top with ½ cup sausage gravy. Serves 5.

Exchanges: ½ meat, 2 breads, ½ milk, 1 fat

~ ~

Cinnamon-Raisin French Toast

4   slices cinnamon-raisin bread
2   eggs, beaten (or ½ c. egg substitute)
⅓   c. nonfat milk
1   tsp. sugar
¼   tsp. vanilla extract
1   tbsp. diet syrup
    Butter-flavored nonstick cooking spray

Combine eggs (or egg substitute), milk, sugar and vanilla in shallow dish; stir well and set aside. Preheat nonstick skillet coated with cooking spray over medium heat. Dip bread slices in egg mixture, turning to coat both sides. Cook 3 to 4 minutes each side or until golden brown. Drizzle each with 1½ teaspoons syrup; serve immediately. Serves 2.
Exchanges: ½ meat, 2 breads, ½ fat (**Omit fat exchange if egg substitute is used.**)

~~~~~~

Cranberry-Cinnamon Scones with Fresh Peaches and Vanilla Cream

1   c. plus 6 tbsp. nonfat milk, divided
1   tbsp. cornstarch
3   tbsp. Splenda sugar substitute, divided
1   tbsp. vanilla extract
1   c. plus 2 tbsp. Bisquick reduced-fat baking mix
2   tbsp. dried cranberries
1   tbsp. sugar
½   tsp. ground cinnamon
⅛   tsp. ground nutmeg
2   tbsp. reduced-calorie margarine, melted
2   c. sliced fresh peaches
    Butter-flavored nonstick cooking spray

Whisk together 1 cup milk, cornstarch and 2 tablespoons Splenda in medium saucepan until well blended. Cook over medium-high heat, stirring constantly until thickened. Remove from heat, stir in vanilla and let cool; transfer vanilla cream to refrigerator to chill.

Preheat oven to 450° F. In large mixing bowl, combine baking mix, cranberries, sugar, remaining Splenda, cinnamon and nutmeg; blend well. Add remaining milk and margarine; stir until just blended. Spoon batter onto nonstick baking sheet coated with cooking spray, creating 4 triangular mounds. Bake 10 to 12 minutes or until lightly browned. Remove from oven and serve each topped with ½ cup sliced peaches and ¼ cup chilled vanilla cream. Serves 4.
Exchanges: 2 breads, ½ fruit, ½ milk, 1 fat

Raspberry-Banana Smoothie

 1 6-oz. container artificially sweetened vanilla-flavored nonfat
    yogurt
 ½ small banana
 ¼ c. raspberries
 ½ c. orange juice

Combine all ingredients in blender; blend well and enjoy! Serves 1.
Exchanges: 2 fruits, 1 milk

~~~~~~

Toasted Bagel and Fresh Fruit

 1 medium whole-wheat bagel, split
 2 tbsp. reduced-fat cream cheese, softened and divided
 ½ small banana, chopped
 ½ c. chopped peaches, canned in juice
 ¼ c. raspberries (fresh or frozen)
 1 c. artificially sweetened vanilla-flavored nonfat yogurt

Toast bagel halves; spread each with 1 tablespoon cream cheese. Set
aside. In small bowl, combine banana, peaches, raspberries and yogurt; mix well and spoon evenly over each bagel half. Serves 2.
Exchanges: 2 breads, 1 fruit, ½ milk, ½ fat

~~~~~~

Turkey Bacon, Potato and Egg Scramble

 2 slices turkey bacon, crisply cooked and crumbled
 ⅓ lb. small red potatoes (about 2 potatoes), cubed
 2 medium eggs, slightly beaten (or ½ c. egg substitute)
 1 c. water
 2 tbsp. nonfat milk
    Dash salt
    Dash pepper
 2 tsp. reduced-calorie margarine
 2 tsp. sliced green onions
 1 tsp. diced pimientos

Bring water and potatoes to boil in small saucepan. Let cook 6 to 8 minutes or until tender; drain and set aside. In small bowl, beat together eggs (or egg substitute), milk, salt and pepper with fork; set aside. Preheat medium skillet over medium-high heat and add margarine. Sauté potatoes 3 to 4 minutes until slightly browned; add green onions and pimientos. Cook 1 minute more, stirring constantly. Pour egg mixture over potato mixture. As the mixture begins to set, gently stir until the uncooked eggs begin to cook and set. Cook 2 to 3 minutes or until eggs are cooked but moist. Sprinkle with crumbled bacon and serve. Serves 2.

Exchanges: 2 breads, ½ fat

☙ LUNCH

Quick and Crunchy Chicken Salad

8 oz. diced cooked chicken breast
1 16-oz. pkg. shredded cabbage with carrots slaw mix
¼ c. sliced red onion
1 3-oz. pkg. ramen noodles, crumbled
½ c. bottled Wish-Bone Citrus Splash vinaigrette salad dressing
1 15-oz. can mandarin orange sections, drained
4 c. chopped romaine lettuce

> **Time-Saving Tip:** No time to bake a chicken? Many grocery stores offer roasted whole chickens in their deli department. Remember to remove the skin before using the chicken for recipes, and keep unused portion refrigerated.

Combine chicken, slaw mix and red onion in large bowl. Add crumbled ramen (save seasoning packet for another use). Pour dressing over top; toss well to coat. Gently stir in mandarin orange sections. Spoon equal amounts onto each of four 1-cup servings of chopped lettuce. Serves 4.

    Serve each with a 1-ounce breadstick.

Exchanges: 2 meats, 1 bread, 2 vegetables, ½ fruit, 1 fat

Taco Pizza

½ lb. extra-lean ground beef
1 medium green bell pepper, diced
1 medium red onion, diced
1 11½-oz. pkg. refrigerated cornbread twists
½ c. prepared salsa (any kind)
1 c. shredded reduced-fat Mexican-blend cheese

Preheat oven to 400° F. In medium nonstick skillet, cook ground beef, bell pepper and onion over medium heat until meat is browned; drain and set aside. Unroll cornbread-twist dough—*but don't separate into strips*. Press dough onto bottom of a 12-inch round pizza pan. Spread salsa evenly over dough; sprinkle with meat mixture and top with cheese. Bake 20 minutes or until crust is browned. Cut into 8 slices. Serves 4.

Serve each with ½ cup Dole tropical fruit cocktail in passion-fruit juice.
Exchanges: 2 meats, 2 breads, 1 vegetable, 1 fruit, 1½ fats

~~~~~~

Long John Silver's

Flavor-baked fish sandwich (no sauce)
Side green beans
Side salad topped with
2 tbsp. low-fat dressing
1 small orange, apple, peach or other fruit
Exchanges: 2 meats, 2 breads, 2 vegetables, 1 fruit, 1 fat

~~~~~~

Turkey-Sausage Noodle Soup

8 oz. cooked smoked turkey sausage, thinly sliced
4 c. water
1 14½-oz. can petite-diced tomatoes with green pepper and onion
1 medium red bell pepper, cut into ½-in. squares
2 3-oz. pkgs. chicken-flavored ramen noodles, crumbled
Black pepper to taste

Combine sausage, water, tomatoes (with liquid), bell pepper and ramen seasoning packets in large saucepan. Bring to boil; add noodles and return to boil 2 to 3 minutes or until noodles are tender. Add pepper to taste. Serves 4.

Serve each with 1 cup carrot sticks and 1 small apple.

Exchanges: 1 ½ meats, 2 breads, 2 vegetables, 1 fruit, 1 fat

~~~~~~

Chic-fil-A Soup and Carrot Salad

1   c. hearty breast of chicken soup
4   saltine crackers
    Small side carrot salad
    Small Icedream cone

Exchanges: 1 meat, 2 breads, 2 vegetables, 1 fruit, 1 fat

~~~~~~

Arby's Chicken Sandwich and Salad

    Light roast chicken deluxe sandwich
    Side garden salad with
2   tbsp. low-fat salad dressing
1   small apple

Exchanges: 2 meats, 2 breads, 2 vegetables, 1 fruit, 1 fat

~~~~~~

Ranch-Style Chicken Fingers

¾   lb. skinless, boneless chicken breasts, cut into thin strips
1 ¾   c. cornflakes crumbs
1   tsp. dried leaf basil
½   c. low-fat buttermilk-ranch salad dressing
    Nonstick cooking spray

Lightly coat a 15x10-inch baking pan with cooking spray; set aside. Preheat oven to 425° F. Combine cornflakes crumbs and basil in shallow dish; mix well and set aside. Place chicken strips in medium bowl; add salad dressing and stir to coat. One at a time, remove chicken strips and roll in crumb mixture. Arrange coated strips on prepared baking pan. Once all strips are arranged on pan, coat lightly with cooking spray. Bake 12 to 15 minutes or until chicken is cooked through. Serves 4.

Serve each with ½ cup prepared marinara and 2 cups salad made of dark greens and low-fat salad dressing.

Exchanges: 2 meats, 2 breads, 2 vegetables, 1 fat

~~~~~~

11-Ounce Healthy Choice Chicken Teriyaki Entreé

1   c. sliced strawberries, tossed with
1   tbsp. prepared poppy seed dressing

Exchanges: 2 meats, 2 breads, 1 vegetable, 1 fruit, 1 fat

~~~~~~

Tex-Mex Salmon-Potato Cakes

2   7.1-oz. pouches Chicken of the Sea skinless, boneless pink salmon
    Hot water
2   c. refrigerated southwestern-style shredded hash brown potatoes
½   c. egg substitute
2   tsp. seafood seasoning
4   tsp. olive oil, divided
¼   c. *Creamy Cocktail Sauce*
    Nonstick cooking spray

> **Time-Saving Tip:** Got a busy week planned? You can make this dish ahead of time and reheat for a quick meal!

Remove fish from pouch; rinse and pat dry with paper towel. Place in large skillet; add just enough water to cover top of fish. Bring to boil; reduce heat to simmer and cook 8 to 10 minutes or until fish begins to flake easily. Remove from skillet; allow to cool slightly. Flake fish into medium bowl; add hash brown potatoes, egg substitute and seafood seasoning; stir gently to combine. Shape mixture into 8 patties and refrigerate 15 to 20 minutes.

When patties are chilled, coat both sides of each with cooking spray; set aside. Preheat large nonstick skillet over medium-high heat; add 2 teaspoons olive oil. Place 4 patties into skillet; cook over medium-high heat 2 to 3 minutes on each side or until browned and heated through. Remove from skillet and keep warm. Add remaining olive oil to skillet and cook remaining patties in same manner. Serve immediately or refrigerate for later use. Serves 4.

Serve each with 1 tablespoon *Creamy Cocktail Sauce* and 1 cup steamed broccoli florets.

Exchanges: 2 meats, 2 breads, 2 vegetables, 1 fat

~ ~

Soup and Sandwich

1 c. Healthy Choice garden vegetable soup
   Peanut-butter sandwich, made with
2 slices diet whole-wheat bread and
1 tbsp. peanut butter
1 small banana

Exchanges: 1 meat, 2 breads, 2 vegetables, 1 fruit, 1 fat

~ ~

Quick and Easy Beef Stew

1 17-oz. pkg. refrigerated Hormel beef tips with gravy
2 10.75-oz. cans Campbell's Healthy Request cream of mushroom soup
1 14½-oz. can petite-diced tomatoes
1 16-oz. pkg. frozen mixed vegetables
1 c. nonfat milk
1 tsp. dried leaf basil

Bring beef tips and gravy, mushroom soup, tomatoes (with liquid), vegetables, milk and basil to boil in large saucepan, stirring occasionally. Serve hot. Serves 4.

Serve each with 1 serving *Kickin' Skillet Cornbread*.

Exchanges: 2½ meats, 2 breads, 2 vegetables, 1½ fats

~ ~

Lean Cuisine Deluxe French Bread Pizza

Serve with 1 serving *Easy Coleslaw*.

Exchanges: 1½ meats, 2½ breads, 1 vegetables, ½ fruit, 1 fat

~ ~

Mediterranean-Style Seafood and Pasta Salad

- 6 oz. cooked salad shrimp
- 1½ c. miniature pasta shells
- 1 c. halved grape tomatoes
- 1 c. diced zucchini
- ½ c. sliced mushrooms
- ¼ c. ripe olives (pits removed)
- 4 oz. Mediterranean-style feta cheese, crumbled
- ½ c. low-fat balsamic vinaigrette salad dressing
- 4 c. fresh spinach leaves

Cook pasta according to package directions, omitting salt and fat. Drain and rinse; place in large bowl. Add shrimp, tomatoes, zucchini, mushrooms, olives and feta cheese; stir to combine. Add salad dressing; toss to coat. Arrange 1 cup spinach leaves on each serving plate; top with shrimp mixture. Serves 4.

Serve each with 1 cup green grapes.

Exchanges: 2 meats, 2 breads, 1 vegetable, 1 fruit, 1 fat

~ ~

Tuna-Veggie Pita Pockets

- 2 6-in. pita bread rounds, cut in half
- 1 6⅛-oz. can chunk tuna packed in water, drained
- ¼ c. low-fat mayonnaise
- ⅛ tsp. black pepper
- 2 tbsp. sweet-pickle relish, drained
- 2 tsp. Dijon mustard
- ½ c. coarsely shredded carrots
- ½ c. finely chopped green bell pepper
- ⅓ c. finely chopped celery
- ⅓ c. thinly sliced green onions, tops only
- 2 c. chopped romaine lettuce
- 4 thick tomato slices

Combine tuna, mayonnaise, black pepper, relish and mustard in large bowl; stir well. Add carrots, bell pepper, celery and green onions; toss gently. Spoon equal amounts of mixture into each pita half. Top each with equal amounts of lettuce and 1 slice tomato. Serves 4.

Serve each with ½ cup canned Dole tropical fruit in juice.
Exchanges: 1 ½ meats, 1 bread, 1 ½ vegetables, 1 fruit, 1 fat

~ ~

Chicken Florentine Muffins with Hollandaise Sauce

8   oz. chopped cooked chicken
4   whole-wheat English muffins, split and toasted
1   10-oz. pkg. frozen creamed spinach
1   1-oz. pkg. hollandaise-sauce mix

Cook spinach in microwave according to package directions; set aside. Prepare hollandaise sauce according to package directions (using reduced-calorie margarine); keep warm. Place chicken into microwave-safe dish and heat in microwave until hot. Spread 1 tablespoon creamed spinach over each muffin half; divide chicken equally over muffin halves and top with 1 tablespoon hollandaise sauce, saving remaining sauce for another use. If necessary, reheat in microwave. Serves 4.

Serve each with 1 cup *Orange-Glazed Carrots and Grapes*.
Exchanges: 2 meats, 2 breads, 2 vegetables, ½ fruit, 1 fat

Creamy Cocktail Sauce

½ c. fat-free sour cream
½ c. fat-free mayonnaise
3 tbsp. seafood cocktail sauce

Combine all ingredients in small bowl; blend well. Keep refrigerated.
Makes about 1¼ cups; serving size is 1 tablespoon.
Exchanges: Free

~~~~~~

Easy Coleslaw

1   16-oz. pkg. shredded cabbage with carrots
1   c. nonfat mayonnaise
¼   c. apple cider vinegar
1   tbsp. honey
1   tsp. celery seeds
¼   c. raisins

Place cabbage mixture in large bowl; set aside. In small bowl, combine
mayonnaise, vinegar and honey; blend well and pour over cabbage.
Toss to coat. Add celery seeds and raisins; toss again. Refrigerate until
ready to serve. Serves 8.
Exchanges: ½ vegetable, ½ fruit

~~~~~~

Kickin' Skillet Cornbread

3   tsp. vegetable oil, divided
1   c. yellow cornmeal
¾   c. all-purpose flour
1½ tsp. baking powder
¼   tsp. baking soda

$\frac{1}{4}$ tsp. salt

$\frac{3}{4}$ c. low-fat buttermilk

1 4-oz. can chopped green chilies, undrained

$\frac{1}{4}$ c. egg substitute

$\frac{1}{2}$ c. frozen whole kernel corn, thawed

Preheat oven to 400° F. Coat 8-inch cast-iron skillet with 1 teaspoon oil; place in oven for 10 minutes. Combine cornmeal, flour, baking powder, baking soda and salt in large bowl; mix well and set aside. In small bowl, combine remaining oil, buttermilk, chilies and egg substitute; mix well and add to cornmeal mixture, stirring until dry ingredients are moistened. Stir in corn; mix well. Spoon into pre-heated skillet; bake 45 minutes or until a wooden pick inserted in center comes out clean. Serves 10.

Exchanges: 1 bread, $\frac{1}{2}$ fat

~~~~~~

Orange-Glazed Carrots and Grapes

2 10-oz. pkgs. frozen whole baby carrots

1 tbsp. brown sugar

2 tsp. cornstarch

$\frac{1}{4}$ tsp. ground ginger

$\frac{1}{8}$ tsp. salt

$\frac{3}{4}$ c. unsweetened orange juice

1 c. seedless red grapes, halved

Cook carrots according to package directions, omitting salt; set aside. Combine brown sugar, cornstarch, ginger and salt in saucepan. Use wire whisk to gradually stir in orange juice; bring to boil over medium heat. Cook 1 minute, stirring constantly; stir in carrots and grapes. Cook 2 minutes more or until heated through, stirring occasionally. Serves 4.

Exchanges: 2 vegetables, $\frac{1}{2}$ fruit

❀ DINNER

Steak with Mushroom Sauce

  2 2-in.-thick beef tenderloin steaks (about 1 lb. total), trimmed of fat
      Salt and pepper to taste
  1 tsp. olive oil
  8 oz. mushrooms, sliced (can use baby portobello and/or button)
  ¼ c. beef consommé
  ¼ c. whipping cream
  2 tsp. Dijon mustard

Season steaks with salt and pepper on both sides; set aside. Preheat oil in large skillet over medium heat; add steaks and cook to desired doneness, turning once (about 10 minutes total for medium-rare and 14 minutes for medium). Transfer steaks to a warm platter. Use same skillet to cook mushrooms 4 minutes over medium heat. Stir in consommé, cream and mustard. Cook and stir over medium heat 2 to 3 minutes or until slightly thickened. Add more seasoning to taste, if desired. Slice each steak into 6 pieces; place 3 pieces on each of 4 plates. Top each with 2 tablespoons mushroom sauce. Serves 4.

    Serve each with 1 *Twice-Baked Broccoli Potato* and a 1-ounce dinner roll.
Exchanges: 3 meats, 2 breads, 1½ vegetables, 1½ fats

~ ~

Cranberry-Apricot Stuffed Chicken Breasts

  4 boneless, skinless chicken breasts (about 1 lb.)
1½ c. herb-seasoned stuffing mix
  ½ c. dried cranberries, divided
  ½ c. apricot all-fruit spread, divided
  ¼ c. reduced-calorie margarine, melted, divided
      Nonstick cooking spray

Preheat oven to 400° F. Place each chicken breast between 2 pieces plastic wrap; pound lightly until breasts are about ¼-inch thick. Discard plastic and set chicken aside. In medium bowl, combine stuffing mix, ¼ cup cranberries, ⅓ cup apricot spread and 3 tablespoons margarine. Stir until moistened; set aside. Combine remaining cranberries, apricot spread and margarine in small bowl; stir well and set aside. Divide stuffing mixture evenly among the four breasts; fold sides of each breast over stuffing and roll up, securing with a toothpick. Place stuffed breasts in 3-quart baking dish coated with cooking spray; bake uncovered 15 minutes. Remove from oven and brush cranberry-apricot glaze mixture over top; bake 10 to 12 minutes more. Serves 4.

Serve each with 1 serving *Veggie Mash.*

Exchanges: 3 meats, 1 bread, 2 vegetables, 1 fruit, 1 fat

~ ~

Pork Chops Dijon

 4 1-in.-thick boneless pork loin chops (about 1 lb.), trimmed of fat
 3 tbsp. Dijon mustard
 2 tbsp. low-fat Italian salad dressing
 $\frac{1}{4}$ tsp. black pepper
 1 medium onion, halved and sliced
     Nonstick cooking spray

Combine mustard, salad dressing and pepper in small bowl; mix well and set aside. Preheat nonstick skillet coated with cooking spray over medium heat. Add chops to skillet and cook 2 minutes on each side. Remove from skillet and set aside. In same skillet, cook onion over medium heat 2 to 3 minutes; push onion to side of skillet and return chops to pan. Spread the mustard mixture over chops; cover skillet and cook over medium-low heat 15 minutes or until meat juices run clear. Spoon onion slices over chops to serve. Serves 4.

Serve each with 1 serving *Vegetable Rice Pilaf,* and 1 cup salad made with dark greens and 2 tablespoons low-fat salad dressing.

Exchanges: 3 meats, 2 breads, 1 $\frac{1}{2}$ vegetables, 1 fat

~ ~

Italian Grilled Chicken

 4 boneless, skinless chicken breasts (about 1 lb.)
 $\frac{3}{4}$ c. low-fat Italian salad dressing

Place chicken breasts and dressing in large sealable plastic bag. Refrigerate 3 hours or overnight. When ready to use, remove breasts from dressing and grill over medium heat 8 minutes; turn and grill 4 to 5 minutes more or until chicken is no longer pink. Serves 4.

Serve each with 1 serving *Grilled Vegetable Kabobs* (including 3 grilled tomatoes) and 1 serving *Garlic Mashed Potatoes*.

Exchanges: 3 meats, 1 bread, 2 vegetables, 1 fat

~~~~~~

Sweet and Sour Chicken with Asian-Style Veggies

    8   boneless, skinless chicken thighs (about 1 lb.)
    2   tsp. olive oil
    1   tsp. five-spice powder, divided (optional)
    ½   c. prepared sweet-and-sour sauce, divided
    1   16-oz. pkg. frozen Oriental stir-fry vegetables
    1   8-oz. can pineapple chunks in juice, drained
    2   tsp. soy sauce
    2   c. cooked brown rice

Preheat oven to 400° F. Arrange chicken thighs in bottom of 3-quart baking dish; brush with olive oil and sprinkle with ½ teaspoon five-spice powder. Bake, uncovered, 20 minutes.

While chicken is cooking, combine remaining five-spice powder, ¼ cup sweet-and-sour sauce, vegetables, pineapple and soy sauce in medium bowl; toss to coat. Remove chicken from oven and push chicken to sides of dish. Brush remaining sweet-and-sour sauce over chicken; arrange vegetable mixture in center of dish. Bake 12 to 15 minutes more, stirring vegetables halfway through. On each serving plate, arrange 1 thigh and 1 cup vegetables over ½ cup brown rice. Serves 4.

Exchanges: 3 meats, 2 breads, 1½ vegetables, ½ fruit, ½ fat

~~~~~~

Bowtie Pasta with Ham and Asparagus

    8   oz. cooked lean ham slices, cut into thin strips
    2   c. bowtie pasta
    1   10-oz. pkg. frozen cut asparagus
    1   8-oz. container reduced-fat soft-style cream cheese with chives and onion

$\frac{1}{3}$ c. nonfat milk

4 tsp. freshly grated Parmesan cheese

Cook pasta according to package directions, omitting salt and oil. During last 5 minutes of cooking time, add asparagus to pasta. Drain and return to pan. In small bowl, combine cream cheese and milk; blend well and set aside. Toss ham with pasta mixture; gently stir in cream-cheese mixture over medium heat until thoroughly heated. Divide evenly among 4 bowls and sprinkle each with 1 teaspoon Parmesan cheese. Serves 4.

Serve each with 1 serving *Green Beans Italiano.*

Exchanges: 3 meats, 2 breads, 2$\frac{1}{2}$ vegetables, 2 fats

~~~~~~

Salmon with Basil Hollandaise

4 5-oz. skinless center-cut salmon fillets

1 10-oz. pkg. hollandaise-sauce mix or

$\frac{1}{2}$ c. prepared hollandaise sauce (can use leftover from *Chicken Florentine Muffins with Hollandaise Sauce*)

1 slice day-old bread, toasted and crumbled

2 tbsp. basil pesto

1 tbsp. freshly grated Parmesan cheese

Nonstick cooking spray

Preheat oven to 425° F. Prepare hollandaise sauce according to package directions, (using reduced-calorie margarine); set aside. Arrange fish on nonstick baking sheet coated with cooking spray; bake 10 to 12 minutes or until fish flakes easily. Combine bread crumbs, hollandaise, pesto and Parmesan cheese in small bowl; stir well and divide mixture evenly over fillets. Return to oven and bake 1 to 2 minutes more. Serves 4.

Serve each with 1 serving each *Roasted Potatoes* and *Dilly Carrots.*

Exchanges: 3 meats, 2 breads, 2 vegetables, 1 fat

~~~~~~

Fish Fillets Florentine au Gratin

4 5-oz. tilapia or other firm white-fish fillets

$\frac{1}{4}$ tsp. lemon-pepper seasoning

1   10-oz. pkg. frozen creamed spinach, thawed
¼   c. fine dry Italian bread crumbs
¼   c. shredded 2% cheddar cheese
    Nonstick cooking spray

Preheat oven to 400° F. Season fillets with lemon-pepper seasoning and arrange on nonstick baking sheet coated with cooking spray; set aside. In small bowl, combine thawed spinach with bread crumbs; spoon mixture evenly over fillets and bake 15 minutes or until fish flakes easily. Top each fillet with 1 tablespoon cheese and bake 1 to 2 minutes more or until cheese is melted. Serves 4.

Serve each with 1 serving *Sweet Potatoes and Sugar Snap Peas*.
Exchanges: 3 meats, 2 breads, 2 vegetables, 1 fat

~~~~~~

Mexican Restaurant Fajitas

½   order chicken or steak fajitas
2   flour tortillas
½   c. refried beans
½   c. salsa
1   tsp. sour cream

Exchanges: 3 to 4 meats, 3 breads, 2 vegetables, 2 fats

~~~~~~

Old-Fashioned Shrimp Boil

1 ½   to 2 lbs. (36 to 40 count) shrimp with shells on, heads off
2   lemons, quartered
2   tbsp. liquid crab boil
2   tbsp. olive oil
1   bay leaf
1   large onion, quartered
2   tbsp. salt
8   small red potatoes, halved
4   small (4-in.) ears corn
4-plus c. water (see directions)
    Ice

Squeeze lemons into large cooking pot. Toss rinds into pan and add liquid crab boil, oil, bay leaf, onion, salt, potatoes and corn. Add enough water to cover mixture; then add 4 more cups water. Bring to boil; continue boiling 5 minutes; add shrimp and continue boiling 2 minutes more. Add enough ice to pot to stop cooking process. Allow to sit 15 minutes; strain and keep warm. Serving size is 9 to 10 shrimp, 4 potato halves and 1 ear corn. Serves 4.

Serve each with ¼ cup *Cocktail Sauce* and 1 serving *Easy Coleslaw* (see Bonus Lunch Recipes).

Exchanges: 3 meats, 2 breads, 1 vegetable, ½ fat

~~~~~~

10-Ounce Lean Cuisine Cheese Lasagna with Chicken Scaloppini Entrée

Serve with 1 cup spinach salad, with sliced tomatoes, sliced mushrooms, 1 teaspoon Bacon Bits and 2 tablespoons reduced-fat French salad dressing, and 4 saltine crackers.

Exchanges: 2½ meats, 2 breads, 2 vegetables, 1 fat

~~~~~~

Turkey Piccata

    1   lb. turkey breast cutlets
    ½   c. low-fat Italian salad dressing, divided
    2   tbsp. low-fat mayonnaise
    2   tsp. finely shredded lemon peel
        Juice from 1 lemon
        Dash black pepper
    1   tbsp. capers, rinsed

Place cutlets and ¼ cup salad dressing into sealable plastic bag; seal and refrigerate 2 to 3 hours or overnight. When ready to use, preheat oven to 425° F and arrange cutlets on nonstick baking sheet. Bake 12 to 15 minutes; remove from oven. In small bowl, combine remaining salad dressing, mayonnaise, lemon peel, lemon juice, black pepper and capers; top each cutlet with 1 tablespoon sauce. Serves 4.

Serve each with 1 serving *Baked Veggie Risotto*.

Exchanges: 3 meats, 2 breads, 1 vegetable, 1 fat

Outback Steakhouse Griller

Chicken-and-veggie or shrimp-and-veggie griller meal, with
House side salad and
2 tbsp. low-fat salad dressing

**Exchanges: (for chicken) 4 meats, 2 breads, 2 vegetables, 2 fats;
(for shrimp) 2 meats, 2 breads, 2 vegetables, 2 fats**

~ ~

Roasted Chicken with Fruit and Pesto

1   3½ to 4½-lb. deli roasted chicken (yields 3½ c. meat)
1   c. apricot all-fruit spread
½   c. dried fruit bits
¼   tsp. ground ginger
½   c. basil pesto

Preheat oven to 350° F. Remove skin from chicken and discard. Strip meat
from bones and place meat in 4-quart baking dish; set aside. In medium
bowl, combine fruit spread, fruit bits, ginger and pesto; stir well and pour
over chicken. Bake 12 to 15 minutes. Serves 6.

Serve each with 1 serving *Roasted Zucchini*, 1 serving *Fruited Saffron Rice*
and 1 wedge *Kickin' Skillet Cornbread* (see Bonus Lunch Recipes).
Exchanges: 3 meats, 2 breads, 1 vegetable, 1 fruit, 1½ fats

Baked Veggie Risotto

    3   c. water
    1   10.75-oz. can condensed Campbell's Healthy Request cream-
        of-chicken soup
    1   c. Arborio or other medium-grain white rice
    ½   c. shredded carrots
    ½   c. diced sweet onion
    1   10-oz. pkg. frozen sugar snap peas
    ¼   tsp. coarsely ground black pepper
    2   tbsp. freshly grated Parmesan cheese

Preheat oven to 375° F. Place water, soup, rice, carrots and onion in
2-quart casserole dish; stir to combine. Bake, covered, 55 minutes;
remove from oven and stir in sugar snap peas and pepper. Cook 5
minutes more; remove from oven and gently stir in cheese. Let
stand 5 minutes before serving. Serves 4.
Exchanges: 2 breads, 1 vegetable

~~~~~~

Cocktail Sauce

    ½   c. no-salt-added tomato sauce
    2   tbsp. minced fresh chives
    2   tbsp. ketchup
    2   tbsp. chili sauce
    1   tbsp. fresh lemon juice
    2   tsp. prepared horseradish
    6   drops Tabasco sauce

In small bowl, combine tomato sauce, chives, ketchup, chili sauce,
lemon juice, horseradish and Tabasco. Serves 4.
Exchanges: Free

Dilly Carrots

  1 lb. baby carrots
  ½ tsp. salt
     Water
  1 tsp. reduced-calorie margarine
  1 tsp. dried dill

Place carrots and salt in medium saucepan; cover with water. Bring to boil and cook 5 minutes or until tender. Drain and return to pan; stir in margarine and dill. Serves 4.
Exchanges: 2 vegetables

~~~~~~

Fruited Saffron Rice

  1 5-oz. pkg. saffron-flavored yellow rice mix
  ½ c. dried fruit bits

Prepare rice according to package directions, adding fruit bits at the beginning. Serves 6.
Exchanges: 2 breads, ½ fruit

~~~~~~

Garlic Mashed Potatoes

  3 c. peeled and cubed baking potatoes
1 to 2 tsp. chopped garlic
     Water
  ¼ c. fat-free half-and-half
  1 tbsp. reduced-calorie margarine
  ¼ tsp. salt
     Dash pepper

Place potatoes and garlic in large saucepan; cover with water and bring to boil. Reduce heat; simmer 20 minutes. Drain and return to pan. Add half-and-half, margarine, salt and pepper to taste. To beat potato mixture, use electric mixer set on medium speed. Serves 4.
Exchanges: 1 bread, ½ fat

Green Beans Italiano

    1   12-oz. pkg. frozen Italian-cut green beans
    1   c. prepared marinara

In medium saucepan, prepare green beans according to package directions; drain and return to pan. Add marinara and heat through over medium heat. Serves 4.

Exchanges: 2 vegetables, ½ fat

~ ~

Grilled Vegetable Kabobs

    5   12- to 14-in. wooden skewers
   12   grape tomatoes
    1   medium yellow squash, cut into 1-in. pieces
    1   medium zucchini, cut into 1-in. pieces
    1   medium red onion, cut into 1-in. pieces
    1   medium red bell pepper, cut into 1-in. pieces
    ¼   c. low-fat Italian salad dressing
        Salt and pepper to taste

Thread all tomatoes onto 1 skewer; set aside. Thread vegetable pieces onto remaining skewers, alternating and using an equal amount of each vegetable for each skewer. Drizzle salad dressing over all skewers and season with salt and pepper. Grill mixed-vegetable kabobs over medium heat 5 to 6 minutes or until tender, turning once. During last 2 to 3 minutes, add tomato kabob to grill. Serves 4 (including 3 tomatoes each serving).

Exchanges: 2 vegetables, ½ fat

~ ~

Roasted Potatoes

  1½   lbs. red potatoes (about 6), each cut into 8 wedges
    2   tsp. olive oil
    ½   tsp. rosemary, crumbled
    ⅛   tsp. pepper
        Nonstick cooking spray

Preheat oven to 450° F. In medium bowl, combine potatoes, oil, rosemary and pepper; toss to coat. Spoon mixture into 2-quart baking dish coated with cooking spray. Bake 40 minutes or until tender, stirring occasionally. Serving size is 12 wedges. Serves 4.

Exchanges: 2 breads, ½ fat

~~~~~~

Roasted Zucchini

    3 lbs. small zucchini
    2 tsp. olive oil
    ½ tsp. dried leaf oregano
    ½ tsp. salt
    ¼ tsp. coarsely ground black pepper

Preheat oven to 450° F. Slice zucchini in half lengthwise; then quarter each half. Toss zucchini pieces with oil, oregano, salt and pepper in large bowl. Arrange in 4-quart baking dish and bake 20 to 25 minutes or until tender. Serves 6.

Exchanges: 1 vegetable

~~~~~~

Sweet Potatoes and Sugar Snap Peas

    2 large sweet potatoes (about 1 lb. each), peeled and cubed
       Water
    1 10-oz. pkg. frozen sugar snap peas, thawed
    ½ tsp. salt, divided
    2 tsp. olive oil
    ½ tsp. dried dill

Cover potatoes with water in medium saucepan; add ¼ teaspoon salt. Bring to boil and simmer 10 to 12 minutes or until potatoes are tender. Drain and set aside, keeping warm. In medium skillet, sauté snap peas in olive oil 3 minutes; stir in dill and remaining salt. Toss peas with potatoes. Serves 4.

Exchanges: 2 breads, 1 vegetable, ½ fat

~~~~~~

Twice-Baked Broccoli Potatoes

2   medium-sized baking potatoes (about ¾ lb.)
2   c. frozen broccoli florets
1   tbsp. low-fat sour cream
1   tbsp. reduced-calorie margarine
    Salt and pepper to taste
1   tbsp. shredded 2% cheddar cheese

Wash potatoes and prick skin several times with fork. Place in microwave-safe dish and microwave on high 5 minutes; turn potatoes over and cook 4 minutes more. Let sit 2 minutes; slice in half lengthwise. Scoop out pulp (being careful not to tear surrounding skin) into medium bowl. Add broccoli, sour cream, margarine, and salt and pepper to taste. Mix well and refill skins with pulp mixture. Top with cheese and microwave 2 to 3 minutes. Serves 4.

Exchanges: 1 bread, 1 vegetable, ½ fat

Vegetable Rice Pilaf

1   c. frozen mixed onion, celery and bell pepper
2   tbsp. reduced-calorie margarine
1   c. brown rice
4   c. reduced-sodium chicken broth
2   c. frozen California-style vegetables, chopped

In large saucepan over medium heat, sauté onion blend in margarine until tender. Add rice and cook until rice is lightly browned. Carefully stir in chicken broth and bring mixture to boil; reduce heat and simmer, covered, 40 minutes. Stir in chopped vegetables and continue simmering 5 minutes more, or until rice is tender and liquid is absorbed. Serves 4.

Exchanges: 2 breads, 1 vegetable, 1 fat

Veggie Mash

3	c. sliced carrots (peel before slicing)
	Water
2	c. coarsely chopped cauliflower
1	c. coarsely chopped broccoli
½	8-oz. container prepared sour cream French onion dip
½	tsp. black pepper

Place carrots in large saucepan; add water to cover. Bring to boil and cook 10 minutes. Add cauliflower and broccoli; cook 3 minutes more. Drain and coarsely mash vegetables; stir in onion dip and black pepper. Serve warm. Serves 4.

Exchanges: 2 vegetables, ½ fat

CONVERSION CHART
EQUIVALENT IMPERIAL AND METRIC MEASUREMENTS

Liquid Measures

Fluid Ounces	U.S.	Imperial	Milliliters
	1 teaspoon	1 teaspoon	5
$\frac{1}{4}$	2 teaspoons	1 dessert spoon	7
$\frac{1}{2}$	1 tablespoon	1 tablespoon	15
1	2 tablespoons	2 tablespoons	28
2	$\frac{1}{4}$ cup	4 tablespoons	56
4	$\frac{1}{2}$ cup or $\frac{1}{4}$ pint		110
5		$\frac{1}{4}$ pint or 1 gill	140
6	$\frac{3}{4}$ cup		170
8	1 cup or $\frac{1}{2}$ pint		225
9			250 or $\frac{1}{4}$ liter
10	$1\frac{1}{4}$ cups	$\frac{1}{2}$ pint	280
12	$1\frac{1}{2}$ cups or $\frac{3}{4}$ pint		340
15		3/4 pint	420
16	2 cups or 1 pint		450
18	$2\frac{1}{4}$ cups		500 or $\frac{1}{2}$ liter
20	$2\frac{1}{2}$ cups	1 pint	560
24	3 cups or $1\frac{1}{2}$ pints		675
25		$1\frac{1}{4}$	700
30	$3\frac{3}{4}$ cups	$1\frac{1}{2}$ pints	840
32	4 cups		900
36	$4\frac{1}{2}$ cups		1,000 or 1 liter
40	5 cups	2 pints or 1 quart	1,120
48	6 cups or 3 pints		1,350
50		$2\frac{1}{2}$ pints	1,400

Solid Measures

U.S. and Imperial Measures		Metric Measures	
Ounces	Pounds	Grams	Kilos
1		28	
2		56	
3½		100	
4	¼	112	
5		140	
6		168	
8	½	225	
9		250	¼
12	¾	340	
16	1	450	
18		500	½
20	1¼	560	
24		675	
27		750	¾
32	2	900	
36	2¼	1,000	1
40	2½	1,100	
48	3	1,350	
54		1,500	1½
64	4	1,800	
72	4½	2,000	2
80	5	2,250	2¼
100	6	2,800	2¾

Oven Temperature Equivalents

Fahrenheit	Celsius	Gas Mark	Description
225	110	$\frac{1}{4}$	Cool
250	130	$\frac{1}{2}$	
275	140	1	Very Slow
300	150	2	
325	170	3	Slow
350	180	4	Moderate
375	190	5	
400	200	6	Moderately Hot
425	220	7	Fairly Hot
450	230	8	Hot
475	240	9	Very Hot
500	250	10	Extremely Hot

LEADER'S DISCUSSION GUIDE

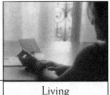

Week One: The God of All Grace

1. Recite this week's memory verse as a group. Ask for two volunteers to recite the verse aloud. Have members form groups of three or four each and share what they've discovered this week about God's promises and their freedom in Christ from Day 1.

2. Read the Nine Commitments and then read Psalm 119:45. Invite members to share within their groups their answers to the question from Day 1 about the prerequisite for walking in freedom; then have them share how following through with their First Place commitments can help them meet their goal of attaining freedom in Christ. Have groups continue to share their answers to questions from Days 1 and 2.

3. Bring the whole group back together, and from Day 3, discuss the important role forgiveness—both seeking and extending it—has in becoming free and transformed in Christ. Continue to discuss the questions from Days 4 and 5.

4. Ask a volunteer to name the six pieces of the armor of God from Ephesians 6:10-18. Discuss the importance of putting on the full armor every day as well as the practical ways that members can use it as they strive to meet their goals in First Place.

5. Invite members to share about a time that they felt the supernatural peace of God during a very difficult time, and have them explain how this peace is profoundly different from other feelings.

6. Close in prayer by inviting five volunteers to pray the Scripture prayers at the end of Days 1 through 5. Finish by praising God for His Word, His promises and His peace, and for meeting the needs of each First Place member.

Week Two: Our Significance to God

1. **Before the meeting**: Draw four columns on a white board, chalkboard or poster board. Above the columns, write the following headings: "God's Love," "God's Rest," "God's Direction" and "God's Provision."

2. Invite a volunteer to recite the memory verse. Have members form groups of three or four each (if possible, use the same small groups from last week) to share what they discovered during week two about their importance to God.

3. With the whole group, read and discuss Matthew 11:28-30. Ask for a show of hands of those who feel they are carrying a heavy burden right now. Assure members that they don't have to share what is burdening them with the group unless they want to do so.

4. Discuss Abraham's ultimate faith that God would provide everything he needed and how this faith was demonstrated in his willingness to sacrifice his son Isaac. Discuss how Abraham and his descendants were blessed because of his obedience and his faith in the Lord's plan for his life.

5. Read Proverbs 2:1-11. Discuss the eight things a person must do in order to gain wisdom, understanding, insight and knowledge. As each is mentioned, discuss how it can be applied in practical ways every day.

6. Direct attention to the board with the four headings. Ask volunteers to share how God displayed Himself this week in one or more of these areas, and write each answer in the appropriate column.

7. Close in prayer by asking for prayer requests especially for those who are carrying burdens, assuring them that they need not share specifics. Invite others to pray for each individual who is especially burdened. Close with phrases of praise to the God who loves us and gives us rest, direction and provision.

Week Three: What Is Grace?

1. As a group, recite this week's memory verse aloud. Ask if there is anyone in the group whose concept of grace has changed since beginning this study or if anybody has any questions about what was covered during weeks one and two.

2. Invite volunteers to name their most precious treasure—besides their family or friends.

3. Read Romans 1:20-23. Discuss why mankind has continually rejected God. Have members share various ways in which we can reject God during our daily lives if we are not making a conscious effort to follow Him in everything we say and do. Is there a difference between a *big* sin and a *small* one?

4. Discuss questions in Day 2, especially pointing out that God's grace is a gift.

5. Invite a volunteer to read Romans 4:13-15. Discuss the questions in the first part of Day 3 up to the scale measuring your amount of faith. Ask volunteers to share when they find it most difficult to have faith. Also discuss the last question in Day 3 about how acting on faith relates to following the Nine Commitments.

6. Invite another volunteer to read Romans 7:14-25. Discuss in what area(s) of their life they identify with Paul and how they combat their temptation. Continue to discuss selected questions in Day 4.

7. Discuss Day 5 questions, especially focusing on the fact that Christians are not condemned. Ask if anyone is suffering from feelings of guilt and if you could pray for each individual right now as a group.

8. Discuss with members their First Place commitment to read the Bible apart from this study. Discuss Day 6 and the benefits of washing your mind and heart with the Word. Refer back to Hebrews 4:12 and discuss what the Word is and what it does for us.

9. Close in prayer. Invite volunteers to pray a prayer of praise for what God's grace means to them.

Week Four: Hindrances to Grace

1. **Before the meeting:** Write the acronym "FEAR" vertically down the left side of a white board, chalkboard or poster board.

2. Invite volunteers to recite last week's memory verse. Ask if anyone can recite the five hindrances to grace that were discussed in this week's study.

3. Direct the group's attention to the board on which the acronym

"FEAR" is written and ask if anyone remembers what the acronym stands for—False Evidence Appearing Real. Complete the acronym by writing the words on the board and ask someone to read 2 Timothy 1:7. Discuss the two kinds of fear mentioned in Day 2.

4. Read James 4:11-12 aloud. With the whole group, discuss the questions from Day 3. Ask volunteers to share a testimony of how they overcame a critical spirit this week.

5. Discuss the questions regarding Luke 23:34 from Day 4; then discuss the question regarding Ephesians 4:26-27. Remind members that an unforgiving heart does more damage to the one who holds on to unforgiveness than to the one who needs to be forgiven. Bitterness will develop in an unforgiving heart, and like acid damages its container, an unforgiving heart will cause damage to the person who won't forgive.

6. Discuss the problems caused by envy and how we can learn to be content with what we have been given in Christ Jesus. Everything in this world will fade away, but as children of God we have been given an inheritance that cannot be matched.

7. Close in prayer, asking for volunteers to pray about each of the five hindrances to grace that were studied this week. Ask if anyone needs prayer for a specific hindrance.

Week Five: The Process of Grace

1. Ask a volunteer to recite this week's memory verse. Discuss how God accepts us just as we are.

2. Discuss with the whole group that we continue to need repentance in our daily lives (from Day 2). Repentance isn't just what you do when you first accept Christ; it must be continually done in order to be consciously aware of and to win the battle over selfish and sinful behaviors that keep us from intimacy with the Lord.

> **Note:** Approach this session prayerfully, as it might be a time to offer members the opportunity to accept Christ as their Savior. Pages 24-25 in the *First Place Leader's Guide* has a simple plan of salvation to aid you, but be open to the Holy Spirit's leading.

3. Remind members what it means to be sanctified (from Day 3) and that keeping their First Place commitments can help them continue the sanctification process spiritually and physically.

4. Have members form small groups to discuss the questions from Day 4. Especially focus on the need to obey and why it is important to be obedient to the Lord even when we don't *feel* like doing so. Invite volunteers to share personal experiences when they learned to obey.

5. Discuss the need for prayer and meditation (from Day 5). It is not enough to know God's Word—you must apply its truths to your life in order to grow into a deeper relationship with God. Invite each member to share which of the psalms listed in the question on the benefits and results of prayer and meditation was especially meaningful and why. Remind members that the commitments of prayer and Bible reading are there to encourage them to spend time daily in prayer and meditation.

6. Close in prayer. Invite members to speak a short sentence prayer thanking God for the lessons of the past week.

Week Six: Attitudes of Grace

1. Recite the memory verse for this week with the whole group. Then read 1 Corinthians 13:4-7 aloud, and discuss what it means to love as Jesus loves and how this passage demonstrates having an attitude of grace. Invite volunteers to share the three phrases from Day 1 that exemplify how Christ has shown His love to them.

2. Invite a volunteer to read Philippians 4:6-7. Discuss the importance of praising and thanking God in all circumstances, even when you might not feel like it. Ask volunteers to share an experience of theirs in which they have received peace and joy from God as a result of praising Him.

3. Form small groups and have them discuss the purpose of suffering in the Christian's life. Instruct them to be prepared to share their group's answers with the whole group. Invite small groups to discuss their answers to the question regarding Colossians 3:12 in Day 3.

4. Bring the whole group back together and ask them to summarize their discussion about the purpose of suffering. Ask for volunteers to share their answers to the last question in Day 4.

5. Read 1 Corinthians 6:12-13. Invite volunteers to share some things that they think are permissible but not beneficial. Point out that these things hinder us from sticking to our First Place commitments. Food is not illegal and it is readily available. In our materialistic society there are also many permissible, even good, things available to distract us from God's ultimate best.

6. Discuss the First Place commitment to fill out the CRs. Remind members that the purpose of the CR is not to point out the things they have not followed through on; rather, it is to serve as an encouragement and a reminder of their goals and their progress toward them.

7. Close in prayer, inviting members to pair off with another member to pray for individual needs. Suggest that they pray for one another in specific areas of struggle with either negative attitudes or with commitments that they are not keeping.

Week Seven: Knowing the God of All Grace

1. **Before the meeting**: On a white board, chalkboard or poster board, write the four different names for God as highlighted in this week's study.

2. Invite a volunteer to recite this week's memory verse. Invite members to try to remember what each name means (without looking in their books) and write the correct meaning beside each name.

3. Discuss the questions for Day 1. Invite one or two volunteers to share how God has shown He is Jehovah-Shammah, "the Lord is there," to them.

4. Invite one or two volunteers to share the prayer they wrote at the end of Day 2. Read Psalm 139 aloud, and invite members to respond to the fact that God is El Roi, "the God who sees."

5. Read Psalm 147:3. Invite volunteers to share a testimony of how Jehovah-Rophi has physically, spiritually or emotionally healed them.

6. Have members form small groups and share about how Jehovah-Jireh has provided for them. Also invite them to share if there is anything that they might be waiting for God to provide. Suggest that each small group pray for members who need perseverance as they wait for God's provision.

7. Invite group members to share with the whole group which verse

particularly spoke to them in the first question of Day 5. Encourage everyone to share which of the four names of God ministered to him or her during this week's study. Invite members to offer a *brief* explanation of why the name they picked stood out.

8. Discuss the First Place commitment to pray and ask volunteers to share how keeping this commitment has helped them in the First Place program and in building their relationship with the Lord.

9. Close in prayer, encouraging sentence prayers of praise and thanksgiving for the God who is always there, the God who sees, the God who heals and the God who provides.

Week Eight: Grace-Filled Men and Women

1. **Before the meeting**: Write the words "humility," "loyalty," "forgiveness," "faithfulness" and "integrity" on a white board, chalkboard or poster board.

2. Invite six members to come forward and have them recite this week's memory verse one phrase at a time with the first person reciting the first phrase (make the breaks at the commas) and the second person reciting the second phrase, and so on. It may take a couple of times before they can say it smoothly.

3. Encourage a volunteer to tell the story of the sinful woman from Day 1. Discuss why her action was a sign of humility.

4. Form small groups to discuss the members' answers to the questions in Day 2. Invite groups to develop a definition of "loyalty" and share it with the whole group.

5. Point out that the focus of Day 3 is not the first time forgiveness has been addressed in this study. Discuss why forgiveness is so important to every aspect of grace and how Hosea is an example of God's grace.

6. Discuss how keeping the First Place commitments demonstrates faithfulness and the importance of keeping your word in every area of your life.

7. Close in prayer, inviting members to pray in their small groups, asking the Lord to help them with their struggles in keeping their commitments.

Week Nine: Extending Grace

1. Recite this week's memory verse as a group. Ask members to raise their hands if they have identified their particular area(s) of spiritual gifting. Discuss the different ways that the same spiritual gift can be used to minister to others, i.e., the gift of teaching could be used in teaching a large group of adults, writing a Bible study, team teaching preschool Sunday School, etc.

2. Discuss Day 1 and Day 2 questions with the whole group, avoiding those that require personal answers.

3. Invite members to share their answers to the questions from Day 3.

4. Form small groups of three or four each and have members share their answers to the questions from Day 4.

5. Explain that assumption and judgment are much the same in that when we assume we know something without finding out the truth, we are making a judgment based on what we assume. Have members discuss in their small groups their answers to the questions from Day 5.

6. Close in prayer. Allow small groups time to share prayer requests; then encourage them to focus on how they might extend grace to others.

Week Ten: Imparting Grace

1. Ask a volunteer to recite this week's memory verse.

2. Discuss the importance of being a follower of Christ, not just acting like one when others are looking. Have members share what it means to *be*, to live your life true to what you believe.

3. Invite volunteers to share their experiences of either being mentored or mentoring someone else. How did each experience impact their life? Discuss with the whole group the question in Day 2 regarding "younger" people mentoring "older" people.

4. Read James 3:1. Invite volunteers to share their answers to the questions in Day 3. Use this opportunity to affirm members that whether they are teaching formally or informally, it is important to teach others about God's love for His children.

Note: As a leader, always be on the lookout for future leaders whom you could raise up. Notice anyone who has special insight into the Word as well as those who are concerned about the needs of others. Is there someone in your group that you might mentor into a future leader?

5. Discuss the process of entrusting and harvesting, and emphasize that we are not the ultimate influence in someone else's life—God is. Entrusting to the Lord those we have mentored and taught and then seeing them stumble can be hard, but we must have faith that God is more than capable of finishing what He started through us. We can be sure that God will harvest the fruit of His good works in others through our dedication to make disciples for the Kingdom.

6. Close in prayer. Spend an extended time in prayer, inviting members to praise the Lord for the work of grace that He has done in their lives during the past 12 weeks. Close by singing "Amazing Grace."

PERSONAL WEIGHT RECORD

Week	Weight	+ or -	Goal This Session	Pounds to Goal
1				
2				
3				
4				
5				
6				
7				
8				
9				
10				
11				
12				
13				
Final				

Beginning Measurements

Waist_____ Hips_____ Thighs_____ Chest_____

Ending Measurements

Waist_____ Hips_____ Thighs_____ Chest_____

COMMITMENT RECORDS

How to Fill Out a Commitment Record

The Commitment Record (CR) is an aid for you in keeping track of your accomplishments. Begin a new CR on the morning of the day your class meets. This ensures that your CR is complete before your next meeting. Turn in the CR weekly to your leader.

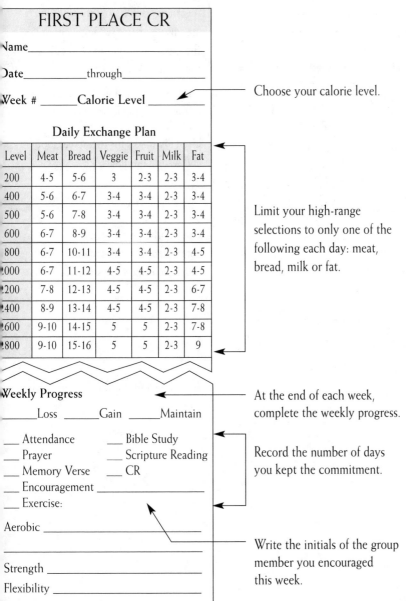

FIRST PLACE CR

Name_____

Date_____through_____

Week # _____Calorie Level _____   Choose your calorie level.

Daily Exchange Plan

Level	Meat	Bread	Veggie	Fruit	Milk	Fat
200	4-5	5-6	3	2-3	2-3	3-4
400	5-6	6-7	3-4	3-4	2-3	3-4
500	5-6	7-8	3-4	3-4	2-3	3-4
600	6-7	8-9	3-4	3-4	2-3	3-4
800	6-7	10-11	3-4	3-4	2-3	4-5
000	6-7	11-12	4-5	4-5	2-3	4-5
200	7-8	12-13	4-5	4-5	2-3	6-7
400	8-9	13-14	4-5	4-5	2-3	7-8
600	9-10	14-15	5	5	2-3	7-8
800	9-10	15-16	5	5	2-3	9

Limit your high-range selections to only one of the following each day: meat, bread, milk or fat.

Weekly Progress   At the end of each week, complete the weekly progress.

_____Loss _____Gain _____Maintain

___ Attendance   ___ Bible Study
___ Prayer   ___ Scripture Reading
___ Memory Verse   ___ CR
___ Encouragement _____
___ Exercise:

Record the number of days you kept the commitment.

Aerobic _____

_____

Strength _____

Flexibility _____

Write the initials of the group member you encouraged this week.

DAY 7: Date _____

Morning _____
_____
_____

Midday _____
_____
_____

Evening _____
_____
_____

Snacks _____
_____
_____

___ Meat _____   ☐ Prayer
___ Bread _____   ☐ Bible Study
___ Vegetable _____   ☐ Scripture Reading
___ Fruit _____   ☐ Memory Verse
___ Milk _____   ☐ Encouragement
___ Fat _____   ☐ Water_____

Exercise
Aerobic _____
_____
Strength _____
Flexibility _____

List the foods you have eaten. On this condensed CR it is not necessary to exchange each food choice. It will be the responsibility of each member that the tally marks you list below are accurate regarding each food choice. If you are unsure of an exchange, check the Live-It section of your copy of the *Member's Guide*.

List the daily food exchange choices to the left of the food groups.

Use tally marks for the actual food and water consumed.

Check off commitments completed. Use tally marks to record each 8-oz. serving of water.

List type and duration of exercise.

FIRST PLACE CR

Name_____

Date_____ through_____
Week # _____ Calorie Level _____

Daily Exchange Plan

Level	Meat	Bread	Veggie	Fruit	Milk	Fat
1200	4-5	5-6	3	2-3	2-3	3-4
1400	5-6	6-7	3-4	3-4	2-3	3-4
1500	5-6	7-8	3-4	3-4	2-3	3-4
1600	6-7	8-9	3-4	3-4	2-3	3-4
1800	6-7	10-11	3-4	3-4	2-3	4-5
2000	6-7	11-12	4-5	4-5	2-3	4-5
2200	7-8	12-13	4-5	4-5	2-3	6-7
2400	8-9	13-14	4-5	4-5	2-3	7-8
2600	9-10	14-15	5	5	2-3	7-8
2800	9-10	15-16	5	5	2-3	9

You may always choose the high range of vegetables and fruits. Limit your high range selections to only one of the following: meat, bread, milk or fat.

Weekly Progress

_____ Loss _____ Gain _____ Maintain

_____ Attendance _____ Bible Study
_____ Prayer _____ Scripture Reading
_____ Memory Verse _____ CR
_____ Encouragement: _____
_____ Exercise _____
Aerobic _____

Strength _____
Flexibility _____

DAY 5: Date_____

Morning_____

Midday_____

Evening_____

Snacks_____

_____ Meat	☐ Prayer
_____ Bread	☐ Bible Study
_____ Vegetable	☐ Scripture Reading
_____ Fruit	☐ Memory Verse
_____ Milk	☐ Encouragement
_____ Fat	_____ Water

Exercise
Aerobic_____

Strength_____
Flexibility_____

DAY 6: Date_____

Morning_____

Midday_____

Evening_____

Snacks_____

_____ Meat	☐ Prayer
_____ Bread	☐ Bible Study
_____ Vegetable	☐ Scripture Reading
_____ Fruit	☐ Memory Verse
_____ Milk	☐ Encouragement
_____ Fat	_____ Water

Exercise
Aerobic_____

Strength_____
Flexibility_____

DAY 7: Date_____

Morning_____

Midday_____

Evening_____

Snacks_____

_____ Meat	☐ Prayer
_____ Bread	☐ Bible Study
_____ Vegetable	☐ Scripture Reading
_____ Fruit	☐ Memory Verse
_____ Milk	☐ Encouragement
_____ Fat	_____ Water

Exercise
Aerobic_____

Strength_____
Flexibility_____

DAY 1: Date_____

Morning_____

Midday_____

Evening_____

Snacks_____

Meat _____	☐ Prayer
Bread _____	☐ Bible Study
Vegetable _____	☐ Scripture Reading
Fruit _____	☐ Memory Verse
Milk _____	☐ Encouragement
Fat _____	Water _____

Exercise
Aerobic _____

Strength _____
Flexibility _____

DAY 2: Date_____

Morning_____

Midday_____

Evening_____

Snacks_____

Meat _____	☐ Prayer
Bread _____	☐ Bible Study
Vegetable _____	☐ Scripture Reading
Fruit _____	☐ Memory Verse
Milk _____	☐ Encouragement
Fat _____	Water _____

Exercise
Aerobic _____

Strength _____
Flexibility _____

DAY 3: Date_____

Morning_____

Midday_____

Evening_____

Snacks_____

Meat _____	☐ Prayer
Bread _____	☐ Bible Study
Vegetable _____	☐ Scripture Reading
Fruit _____	☐ Memory Verse
Milk _____	☐ Encouragement
Fat _____	Water _____

Exercise
Aerobic _____

Strength _____
Flexibility _____

DAY 4: Date_____

Morning_____

Midday_____

Evening_____

Snacks_____

Meat _____	☐ Prayer
Bread _____	☐ Bible Study
Vegetable _____	☐ Scripture Reading
Fruit _____	☐ Memory Verse
Milk _____	☐ Encouragement
Fat _____	Water _____

Exercise
Aerobic _____

Strength _____
Flexibility _____

FIRST PLACE CR

Name _____

Date _____ through _____

Week # _____ Calorie Level _____

Daily Exchange Plan

Level	Meat	Bread	Veggie	Fruit	Milk	Fat
1200	4-5	5-6	3	2-3	2-3	3-4
1400	5-6	6-7	3-4	3-4	2-3	3-4
1500	5-6	7-8	3-4	3-4	2-3	3-4
1600	6-7	8-9	3-4	3-4	2-3	3-4
1800	6-7	10-11	3-4	3-4	2-3	4-5
2000	6-7	11-12	4-5	4-5	2-3	4-5
2200	7-8	12-13	4-5	4-5	2-3	6-7
2400	8-9	13-14	4-5	4-5	2-3	7-8
2600	9-10	14-15	5	5	2-3	7-8
2800	9-10	15-16	5	5	2-3	9

You may always choose the high range of vegetables and fruits. Limit your high range selections to only one of the following: meat, bread, milk or fat.

Weekly Progress

_____ Loss _____ Gain _____ Maintain

_____ Attendance _____ Bible Study
_____ Prayer _____ Scripture Reading
_____ Memory Verse _____ CR
_____ Encouragement:
_____ Exercise
Aerobic _____

Strength _____
Flexibility _____

DAY 5: Date _____

Morning _____

Midday _____

Evening _____

Snacks _____

_____ Meat   ☐ Prayer
_____ Bread   ☐ Bible Study
_____ Vegetable   ☐ Scripture Reading
_____ Fruit   ☐ Memory Verse
_____ Milk   ☐ Encouragement
_____ Fat   _____ Water

Exercise
Aerobic _____

Strength _____
Flexibility _____

DAY 6: Date _____

Morning _____

Midday _____

Evening _____

Snacks _____

_____ Meat   ☐ Prayer
_____ Bread   ☐ Bible Study
_____ Vegetable   ☐ Scripture Reading
_____ Fruit   ☐ Memory Verse
_____ Milk   ☐ Encouragement
_____ Fat   _____ Water

Exercise
Aerobic _____

Strength _____
Flexibility _____

DAY 7: Date _____

Morning _____

Midday _____

Evening _____

Snacks _____

_____ Meat   ☐ Prayer
_____ Bread   ☐ Bible Study
_____ Vegetable   ☐ Scripture Reading
_____ Fruit   ☐ Memory Verse
_____ Milk   ☐ Encouragement
_____ Fat   _____ Water

Exercise
Aerobic _____

Strength _____
Flexibility _____

DAY 1: Date _____

Morning _____

Midday _____

Evening _____

Snacks _____

___ Meat ___ ☐ Prayer
___ Bread ___ ☐ Bible Study
___ Vegetable ___ ☐ Scripture Reading
___ Fruit ___ ☐ Memory Verse
___ Milk ___ ☐ Encouragement
___ Fat ___ Water ___

Exercise
Aerobic _____
Strength _____
Flexibility _____

DAY 2: Date _____

Morning _____

Midday _____

Evening _____

Snacks _____

___ Meat ___ ☐ Prayer
___ Bread ___ ☐ Bible Study
___ Vegetable ___ ☐ Scripture Reading
___ Fruit ___ ☐ Memory Verse
___ Milk ___ ☐ Encouragement
___ Fat ___ Water ___

Exercise
Aerobic _____
Strength _____
Flexibility _____

DAY 3: Date _____

Morning _____

Midday _____

Evening _____

Snacks _____

___ Meat ___ ☐ Prayer
___ Bread ___ ☐ Bible Study
___ Vegetable ___ ☐ Scripture Reading
___ Fruit ___ ☐ Memory Verse
___ Milk ___ ☐ Encouragement
___ Fat ___ Water ___

Exercise
Aerobic _____
Strength _____
Flexibility _____

DAY 4: Date _____

Morning _____

Midday _____

Evening _____

Snacks _____

___ Meat ___ ☐ Prayer
___ Bread ___ ☐ Bible Study
___ Vegetable ___ ☐ Scripture Reading
___ Fruit ___ ☐ Memory Verse
___ Milk ___ ☐ Encouragement
___ Fat ___ Water ___

Exercise
Aerobic _____
Strength _____
Flexibility _____

FIRST PLACE CR

Name _____
Date _____ through _____
Week # _____ Calorie Level _____

Daily Exchange Plan

Level	Meat	Bread	Veggie	Fruit	Milk	Fat
1200	4-5	5-6	3	2-3	2-3	3-4
1400	5-6	6-7	3-4	3-4	2-3	3-4
1500	5-6	7-8	3-4	3-4	2-3	3-4
1600	6-7	8-9	3-4	3-4	2-3	3-4
1800	6-7	10-11	3-4	3-4	2-3	4-5
2000	6-7	11-12	4-5	4-5	2-3	4-5
2200	7-8	12-13	4-5	4-5	2-3	6-7
2400	8-9	13-14	4-5	4-5	2-3	7-8
2600	9-10	14-15	5	5	2-3	7-8
2800	9-10	15-16	5	5	2-3	9

You may always choose the high range of vegetables and fruits. Limit your high range selections to only one of the following: meat, bread, milk or fat.

Weekly Progress

_____ Loss _____ Gain _____ Maintain

_____ Attendance _____ Bible Study
_____ Prayer _____ Scripture Reading
_____ Memory Verse _____ CR
_____ Encouragement:
_____ Exercise
Aerobic _____

Strength _____
Flexibility _____

DAY 5: Date _____

Morning _____
_____

Midday _____
_____
_____

Evening _____
_____

Snacks _____
_____

_____ Meat ☐ Prayer
_____ Bread ☐ Bible Study
_____ Vegetable ☐ Scripture Reading
_____ Fruit ☐ Memory Verse
_____ Milk ☐ Encouragement
_____ Fat Water _____

Exercise
Aerobic _____

Strength _____
Flexibility _____

DAY 6: Date _____

Morning _____
_____

Midday _____
_____
_____

Evening _____
_____

Snacks _____
_____

_____ Meat ☐ Prayer
_____ Bread ☐ Bible Study
_____ Vegetable ☐ Scripture Reading
_____ Fruit ☐ Memory Verse
_____ Milk ☐ Encouragement
_____ Fat Water _____

Exercise
Aerobic _____

Strength _____
Flexibility _____

DAY 7: Date _____

Morning _____
_____

Midday _____
_____
_____

Evening _____
_____

Snacks _____
_____

_____ Meat ☐ Prayer
_____ Bread ☐ Bible Study
_____ Vegetable ☐ Scripture Reading
_____ Fruit ☐ Memory Verse
_____ Milk ☐ Encouragement
_____ Fat Water _____

Exercise
Aerobic _____

Strength _____
Flexibility _____

DAY 1: Date_____

Morning _____

Midday _____

Evening _____

Snacks _____

____ Meat   □ Prayer
____ Bread   □ Bible Study
____ Vegetable   □ Scripture Reading
____ Fruit   □ Memory Verse
____ Milk   □ Encouragement
____ Fat   □ Water

Exercise
Aerobic _____
Strength _____
Flexibility _____

DAY 2: Date_____

Morning _____

Midday _____

Evening _____

Snacks _____

____ Meat   □ Prayer
____ Bread   □ Bible Study
____ Vegetable   □ Scripture Reading
____ Fruit   □ Memory Verse
____ Milk   □ Encouragement
____ Fat   □ Water

Exercise
Aerobic _____
Strength _____
Flexibility _____

DAY 3: Date_____

Morning _____

Midday _____

Evening _____

Snacks _____

____ Meat   □ Prayer
____ Bread   □ Bible Study
____ Vegetable   □ Scripture Reading
____ Fruit   □ Memory Verse
____ Milk   □ Encouragement
____ Fat   □ Water

Exercise
Aerobic _____
Strength _____
Flexibility _____

DAY 4: Date_____

Morning _____

Midday _____

Evening _____

Snacks _____

____ Meat   □ Prayer
____ Bread   □ Bible Study
____ Vegetable   □ Scripture Reading
____ Fruit   □ Memory Verse
____ Milk   □ Encouragement
____ Fat   □ Water

Exercise
Aerobic _____
Strength _____
Flexibility _____

FIRST PLACE CR

Name _____

Date _____ through _____

Week # _____ Calorie Level _____

Daily Exchange Plan

Level	Meat	Bread	Veggie	Fruit	Milk	Fat
1200	4-5	5-6	3	2-3	2-3	3-4
1400	5-6	6-7	3-4	3-4	2-3	3-4
1500	5-6	7-8	3-4	3-4	2-3	3-4
1600	6-7	8-9	3-4	3-4	2-3	3-4
1800	6-7	10-11	3-4	3-4	2-3	4-5
2000	6-7	11-12	4-5	4-5	2-3	4-5
2200	7-8	12-13	4-5	4-5	2-3	6-7
2400	8-9	13-14	4-5	4-5	2-3	7-8
2600	9-10	14-15	5	5	2-3	7-8
2800	9-10	15-16	5	5	2-3	9

You may always choose the high range of vegetables and fruits. Limit your high range selections to only one of the following: meat, bread, milk or fat.

Weekly Progress

_____ Loss _____ Gain _____ Maintain

_____ Attendance   _____ Bible Study
_____ Prayer   _____ Scripture Reading
_____ Memory Verse   _____ CR
_____ Encouragement:
_____ Exercise
Aerobic

Strength
Flexibility

DAY 5: Date _____

Morning _____

Midday _____

Evening _____

Snacks _____

_____ Meat   ☐ Prayer
_____ Bread   ☐ Bible Study
_____ Vegetable   ☐ Scripture Reading
_____ Fruit   ☐ Memory Verse
_____ Milk   ☐ Encouragement
_____ Fat   _____ Water

Exercise
Aerobic _____

Strength _____
Flexibility _____

DAY 6: Date _____

Morning _____

Midday _____

Evening _____

Snacks _____

_____ Meat   ☐ Prayer
_____ Bread   ☐ Bible Study
_____ Vegetable   ☐ Scripture Reading
_____ Fruit   ☐ Memory Verse
_____ Milk   ☐ Encouragement
_____ Fat   _____ Water

Exercise
Aerobic _____

Strength _____
Flexibility _____

DAY 7: Date _____

Morning _____

Midday _____

Evening _____

Snacks _____

_____ Meat   ☐ Prayer
_____ Bread   ☐ Bible Study
_____ Vegetable   ☐ Scripture Reading
_____ Fruit   ☐ Memory Verse
_____ Milk   ☐ Encouragement
_____ Fat   _____ Water

Exercise
Aerobic _____

Strength _____
Flexibility _____

DAY 1: Date _____

Morning _____

Midday _____

Evening _____

Snacks _____

___ Meat   ☐ Prayer
___ Bread   ☐ Bible Study
___ Vegetable   ☐ Scripture Reading
___ Fruit   ☐ Memory Verse
___ Milk   ☐ Encouragement
___ Fat   ___ Water

Exercise
Aerobic _____
Strength _____
Flexibility _____

DAY 2: Date _____

Morning _____

Midday _____

Evening _____

Snacks _____

___ Meat   ☐ Prayer
___ Bread   ☐ Bible Study
___ Vegetable   ☐ Scripture Reading
___ Fruit   ☐ Memory Verse
___ Milk   ☐ Encouragement
___ Fat   ___ Water

Exercise
Aerobic _____
Strength _____
Flexibility _____

DAY 3: Date _____

Morning _____

Midday _____

Evening _____

Snacks _____

___ Meat   ☐ Prayer
___ Bread   ☐ Bible Study
___ Vegetable   ☐ Scripture Reading
___ Fruit   ☐ Memory Verse
___ Milk   ☐ Encouragement
___ Fat   ___ Water

Exercise
Aerobic _____
Strength _____
Flexibility _____

DAY 4: Date _____

Morning _____

Midday _____

Evening _____

Snacks _____

___ Meat   ☐ Prayer
___ Bread   ☐ Bible Study
___ Vegetable   ☐ Scripture Reading
___ Fruit   ☐ Memory Verse
___ Milk   ☐ Encouragement
___ Fat   ___ Water

Exercise
Aerobic _____
Strength _____
Flexibility _____

FIRST PLACE CR

Name _____

Date _____ through _____

Week # _____   Calorie Level _____

Daily Exchange Plan

Level	Meat	Bread	Veggie	Fruit	Milk	Fat
1200	4-5	5-6	3	2-3	2-3	3-4
1400	5-6	6-7	3-4	3-4	2-3	3-4
1500	5-6	7-8	3-4	3-4	2-3	3-4
1600	6-7	8-9	3-4	3-4	2-3	3-4
1800	6-7	10-11	3-4	3-4	2-3	4-5
2000	6-7	11-12	4-5	4-5	2-3	4-5
2200	7-8	12-13	4-5	4-5	2-3	6-7
2400	8-9	13-14	4-5	4-5	2-3	7-8
2600	9-10	14-15	5	5	2-3	7-8
2800	9-10	15-16	5	5	2-3	9

You may always choose the high range of vegetables and fruits. Limit your high range selections to only one of the following: meat, bread, milk or fat.

Weekly Progress

___ Loss ___ Gain ___ Maintain

___ Attendance
___ Prayer
___ Memory Verse
___ Encouragement:
___ Exercise
Aerobic

___ Bible Study
___ Scripture Reading
___ CR

Strength _____
Flexibility _____

DAY 5: Date _____

Morning _____

Midday _____

Evening _____

Snacks _____

___ Meat
___ Bread
___ Vegetable
___ Fruit
___ Milk
___ Fat

☐ Prayer
☐ Bible Study
☐ Scripture Reading
☐ Memory Verse
☐ Encouragement
☐ Water

Exercise
Aerobic _____

Strength _____
Flexibility _____

DAY 6: Date _____

Morning _____

Midday _____

Evening _____

Snacks _____

___ Meat
___ Bread
___ Vegetable
___ Fruit
___ Milk
___ Fat

☐ Prayer
☐ Bible Study
☐ Scripture Reading
☐ Memory Verse
☐ Encouragement
☐ Water

Exercise
Aerobic _____

Strength _____
Flexibility _____

DAY 7: Date _____

Morning _____

Midday _____

Evening _____

Snacks _____

___ Meat
___ Bread
___ Vegetable
___ Fruit
___ Milk
___ Fat

☐ Prayer
☐ Bible Study
☐ Scripture Reading
☐ Memory Verse
☐ Encouragement
☐ Water

Exercise
Aerobic _____

Strength _____
Flexibility _____

DAY 1: Date _____

Morning _____

Midday _____

Evening _____

Snacks _____

___ Meat	☐ Prayer
___ Bread	☐ Bible Study
___ Vegetable	☐ Scripture Reading
___ Fruit	☐ Memory Verse
___ Milk	☐ Encouragement
___ Fat ___ Water ___	

Exercise
Aerobic _____
Strength _____
Flexibility _____

DAY 2: Date _____

Morning _____

Midday _____

Evening _____

Snacks _____

___ Meat	☐ Prayer
___ Bread	☐ Bible Study
___ Vegetable	☐ Scripture Reading
___ Fruit	☐ Memory Verse
___ Milk	☐ Encouragement
___ Fat ___ Water ___	

Exercise
Aerobic _____
Strength _____
Flexibility _____

DAY 3: Date _____

Morning _____

Midday _____

Evening _____

Snacks _____

___ Meat	☐ Prayer
___ Bread	☐ Bible Study
___ Vegetable	☐ Scripture Reading
___ Fruit	☐ Memory Verse
___ Milk	☐ Encouragement
___ Fat ___ Water ___	

Exercise
Aerobic _____
Strength _____
Flexibility _____

DAY 4: Date _____

Morning _____

Midday _____

Evening _____

Snacks _____

___ Meat	☐ Prayer
___ Bread	☐ Bible Study
___ Vegetable	☐ Scripture Reading
___ Fruit	☐ Memory Verse
___ Milk	☐ Encouragement
___ Fat ___ Water ___	

Exercise
Aerobic _____
Strength _____
Flexibility _____

FIRST PLACE CR

Name _____

Date _____ through _____

Week # _____ Calorie Level _____

Daily Exchange Plan

Level	Meat	Bread	Veggie	Fruit	Milk	Fat
1200	4-5	5-6	3	2-3	2-3	3-4
1400	5-6	6-7	3-4	3-4	2-3	3-4
1500	5-6	7-8	3-4	3-4	2-3	3-4
1600	6-7	8-9	3-4	3-4	2-3	3-4
1800	6-7	10-11	3-4	3-4	2-3	4-5
2000	6-7	11-12	4-5	4-5	2-3	4-5
2200	7-8	12-13	4-5	4-5	2-3	6-7
2400	8-9	13-14	4-5	4-5	2-3	7-8
2600	9-10	14-15	5	5	2-3	7-8
2800	9-10	15-16	5	5	2-3	9

You may always choose the high range of vegetables and fruits. Limit your high range selections to only one of the following: meat, bread, milk or fat.

Weekly Progress

_____ Loss _____ Gain _____ Maintain

_____ Attendance _____ Bible Study
_____ Prayer _____ Scripture Reading
_____ Memory Verse _____ CR
_____ Encouragement:
_____ Exercise
Aerobic _____

Strength _____
Flexibility _____

DAY 5: Date _____

Morning _____

Midday _____

Evening _____

Snacks _____

_____ Meat   ☐ Prayer
_____ Bread   ☐ Bible Study
_____ Vegetable ☐ Scripture Reading
_____ Fruit   ☐ Memory Verse
_____ Milk   ☐ Encouragement
_____ Fat   _____ Water
Exercise
Aerobic _____

Strength _____
Flexibility _____

DAY 6: Date _____

Morning _____

Midday _____

Evening _____

Snacks _____

_____ Meat   ☐ Prayer
_____ Bread   ☐ Bible Study
_____ Vegetable ☐ Scripture Reading
_____ Fruit   ☐ Memory Verse
_____ Milk   ☐ Encouragement
_____ Fat   _____ Water
Exercise
Aerobic _____

Strength _____
Flexibility _____

DAY 7: Date _____

Morning _____

Midday _____

Evening _____

Snacks _____

_____ Meat   ☐ Prayer
_____ Bread   ☐ Bible Study
_____ Vegetable ☐ Scripture Reading
_____ Fruit   ☐ Memory Verse
_____ Milk   ☐ Encouragement
_____ Fat   _____ Water
Exercise
Aerobic _____

Strength _____
Flexibility _____

DAY 1: Date _____

Morning _____

Midday _____

Evening _____

Snacks _____

Meat _____	☐ Prayer
Bread _____	☐ Bible Study
Vegetable _____	☐ Scripture Reading
Fruit _____	☐ Memory Verse
Milk _____	☐ Encouragement
Fat _____ Water _____	

Exercise
Aerobic _____
Strength _____
Flexibility _____

DAY 2: Date _____

Morning _____

Midday _____

Evening _____

Snacks _____

Meat _____	☐ Prayer
Bread _____	☐ Bible Study
Vegetable _____	☐ Scripture Reading
Fruit _____	☐ Memory Verse
Milk _____	☐ Encouragement
Fat _____ Water _____	

Exercise
Aerobic _____
Strength _____
Flexibility _____

DAY 3: Date _____

Morning _____

Midday _____

Evening _____

Snacks _____

Meat _____	☐ Prayer
Bread _____	☐ Bible Study
Vegetable _____	☐ Scripture Reading
Fruit _____	☐ Memory Verse
Milk _____	☐ Encouragement
Fat _____ Water _____	

Exercise
Aerobic _____
Strength _____
Flexibility _____

DAY 4: Date _____

Morning _____

Midday _____

Evening _____

Snacks _____

Meat _____	☐ Prayer
Bread _____	☐ Bible Study
Vegetable _____	☐ Scripture Reading
Fruit _____	☐ Memory Verse
Milk _____	☐ Encouragement
Fat _____ Water _____	

Exercise
Aerobic _____
Strength _____
Flexibility _____

FIRST PLACE CR

Name _____

Date _____ through _____

Week # _____ Calorie Level _____

Daily Exchange Plan

Level	Meat	Bread	Veggie	Fruit	Milk	Fat
1200	4-5	5-6	3	2-3	2-3	3-4
1400	5-6	6-7	3-4	3-4	2-3	3-4
1500	5-6	7-8	3-4	3-4	2-3	3-4
1600	6-7	8-9	3-4	3-4	2-3	3-4
1800	6-7	10-11	3-4	3-4	2-3	3-4
2000	6-7	11-12	4-5	4-5	2-3	4-5
2200	7-8	12-13	4-5	4-5	2-3	4-5
2400	8-9	13-14	4-5	4-5	2-3	6-7
2600	9-10	14-15	5	5	2-3	7-8
2800	9-10	15-16	5	5	2-3	9

You may always choose the high range of vegetables and fruits. Limit your high range selections to only one of the following: meat, bread, milk or fat.

Weekly Progress

_____ Loss _____ Gain _____ Maintain

_____ Attendance _____ Bible Study
_____ Prayer _____ Scripture Reading
_____ Memory Verse _____ CR
_____ Encouragement: _____
_____ Exercise
Aerobic _____
Strength _____
Flexibility _____

DAY 5: Date _____

Morning _____

Midday _____

Evening _____

Snacks _____

Meat _____	□ Prayer
Bread _____	□ Bible Study
Vegetable _____	□ Scripture Reading
Fruit _____	□ Memory Verse
Milk _____	□ Encouragement
Fat _____	□ Water

Exercise
Aerobic _____

Strength _____
Flexibility _____

DAY 6: Date _____

Morning _____

Midday _____

Evening _____

Snacks _____

Meat _____	□ Prayer
Bread _____	□ Bible Study
Vegetable _____	□ Scripture Reading
Fruit _____	□ Memory Verse
Milk _____	□ Encouragement
Fat _____	□ Water

Exercise
Aerobic _____

Strength _____
Flexibility _____

DAY 7: Date _____

Morning _____

Midday _____

Evening _____

Snacks _____

Meat _____	□ Prayer
Bread _____	□ Bible Study
Vegetable _____	□ Scripture Reading
Fruit _____	□ Memory Verse
Milk _____	□ Encouragement
Fat _____	□ Water

Exercise
Aerobic _____

Strength _____
Flexibility _____

DAY 1: Date _____

Morning _____

Midday _____

Evening _____

Snacks _____

___ Meat	☐ Prayer
___ Bread	☐ Bible Study
___ Vegetable	☐ Scripture Reading
___ Fruit	☐ Memory Verse
___ Milk	☐ Encouragement
___ Fat	___ Water

Exercise
Aerobic _____
Strength _____
Flexibility _____

DAY 2: Date _____

Morning _____

Midday _____

Evening _____

Snacks _____

___ Meat	☐ Prayer
___ Bread	☐ Bible Study
___ Vegetable	☐ Scripture Reading
___ Fruit	☐ Memory Verse
___ Milk	☐ Encouragement
___ Fat	___ Water

Exercise
Aerobic _____
Strength _____
Flexibility _____

DAY 3: Date _____

Morning _____

Midday _____

Evening _____

Snacks _____

___ Meat	☐ Prayer
___ Bread	☐ Bible Study
___ Vegetable	☐ Scripture Reading
___ Fruit	☐ Memory Verse
___ Milk	☐ Encouragement
___ Fat	___ Water

Exercise
Aerobic _____
Strength _____
Flexibility _____

DAY 4: Date _____

Morning _____

Midday _____

Evening _____

Snacks _____

___ Meat	☐ Prayer
___ Bread	☐ Bible Study
___ Vegetable	☐ Scripture Reading
___ Fruit	☐ Memory Verse
___ Milk	☐ Encouragement
___ Fat	___ Water

Exercise
Aerobic _____
Strength _____
Flexibility _____

FIRST PLACE CR

Name _____

Date _____ through _____

Week # _____ Calorie Level _____

Daily Exchange Plan

Level	Meat	Bread	Veggie	Fruit	Milk	Fat
1200	4-5	5-6	3	2-3	2-3	3-4
1400	5-6	6-7	3-4	3-4	2-3	3-4
1500	5-6	7-8	3-4	3-4	2-3	3-4
1600	6-7	8-9	3-4	3-4	2-3	3-4
1800	6-7	10-11	3-4	3-4	2-3	4-5
2000	6-7	11-12	4-5	4-5	2-3	4-5
2200	7-8	12-13	4-5	4-5	2-3	6-7
2400	8-9	13-14	4-5	4-5	2-3	7-8
2600	9-10	14-15	5	5	2-3	7-8
2800	9-10	15-16	5	5	2-3	9

You may always choose the high range of vegetables and fruits. Limit your high range selections to only one of the following: meat, bread, milk or fat.

Weekly Progress

_____ Loss _____ Gain _____ Maintain

_____ Attendance _____ Bible Study
_____ Prayer _____ Scripture Reading
_____ Memory Verse _____ CR
_____ Encouragement:
_____ Exercise
Aerobic _____

Strength _____
Flexibility _____

DAY 5: Date _____

Morning _____

Midday _____

Evening _____

Snacks _____

_____ Meat ☐ Prayer
_____ Bread ☐ Bible Study
_____ Vegetable ☐ Scripture Reading
_____ Fruit ☐ Memory Verse
_____ Milk ☐ Encouragement
_____ Fat _____ Water

Exercise
Aerobic _____

Strength _____
Flexibility _____

DAY 6: Date _____

Morning _____

Midday _____

Evening _____

Snacks _____

_____ Meat ☐ Prayer
_____ Bread ☐ Bible Study
_____ Vegetable ☐ Scripture Reading
_____ Fruit ☐ Memory Verse
_____ Milk ☐ Encouragement
_____ Fat _____ Water

Exercise
Aerobic _____

Strength _____
Flexibility _____

DAY 7: Date _____

Morning _____

Midday _____

Evening _____

Snacks _____

_____ Meat ☐ Prayer
_____ Bread ☐ Bible Study
_____ Vegetable ☐ Scripture Reading
_____ Fruit ☐ Memory Verse
_____ Milk ☐ Encouragement
_____ Fat _____ Water

Exercise
Aerobic _____

Strength _____
Flexibility _____

DAY 1: Date _____

Morning _____

Midday _____

Evening _____

Snacks _____

_____ Meat   ☐ Prayer
_____ Bread   ☐ Bible Study
_____ Vegetable   ☐ Scripture Reading
_____ Fruit   ☐ Memory Verse
_____ Milk   ☐ Encouragement
_____ Fat   _____ Water

Exercise
Aerobic _____
Strength _____
Flexibility _____

DAY 2: Date _____

Morning _____

Midday _____

Evening _____

Snacks _____

_____ Meat   ☐ Prayer
_____ Bread   ☐ Bible Study
_____ Vegetable   ☐ Scripture Reading
_____ Fruit   ☐ Memory Verse
_____ Milk   ☐ Encouragement
_____ Fat   _____ Water

Exercise
Aerobic _____
Strength _____
Flexibility _____

DAY 3: Date _____

Morning _____

Midday _____

Evening _____

Snacks _____

_____ Meat   ☐ Prayer
_____ Bread   ☐ Bible Study
_____ Vegetable   ☐ Scripture Reading
_____ Fruit   ☐ Memory Verse
_____ Milk   ☐ Encouragement
_____ Fat   _____ Water

Exercise
Aerobic _____
Strength _____
Flexibility _____

DAY 4: Date _____

Morning _____

Midday _____

Evening _____

Snacks _____

_____ Meat   ☐ Prayer
_____ Bread   ☐ Bible Study
_____ Vegetable   ☐ Scripture Reading
_____ Fruit   ☐ Memory Verse
_____ Milk   ☐ Encouragement
_____ Fat   _____ Water

Exercise
Aerobic _____
Strength _____
Flexibility _____

DAY 5: Date _____   **DAY 6:** Date _____   **DAY 7:** Date _____

FIRST PLACE CR

Name _____

Date _____ through _____

Week # _____ Calorie Level _____

Daily Exchange Plan

Level	Meat	Bread	Veggie	Fruit	Milk	Fat
1200	4-5	5-6	3	2-3	2-3	3-4
1400	5-6	6-7	3-4	3-4	2-3	3-4
1500	5-6	7-8	3-4	3-4	2-3	3-4
1600	6-7	8-9	3-4	3-4	2-3	3-4
1800	6-7	10-11	3-4	3-4	2-3	4-5
2000	6-7	11-12	4-5	4-5	2-3	4-5
2200	7-8	12-13	4-5	4-5	2-3	6-7
2400	8-9	13-14	4-5	4-5	2-3	7-8
2600	9-10	14-15	5	5	2-3	7-8
2800	9-10	15-16	5	5	2-3	9

You may always choose the high range of vegetables and fruits. Limit your high range selections to only one of the following: meat, bread, milk or fat.

Weekly Progress

_____ Loss _____ Gain _____ Maintain

_____ Attendance   _____ Bible Study

_____ Prayer   _____ Scripture Reading

_____ Memory Verse   _____ CR

_____ Encouragement:

_____ Exercise

Aerobic _____

Strength _____

Flexibility _____

Morning _____

Midday _____

Evening _____

Snacks _____

_____ Meat   ☐ Prayer

_____ Bread   ☐ Bible Study

_____ Vegetable   ☐ Scripture Reading

_____ Fruit   ☐ Memory Verse

_____ Milk   ☐ Encouragement

_____ Fat   _____ Water

Exercise

Aerobic _____

Strength _____

Flexibility _____

Morning _____

Midday _____

Evening _____

Snacks _____

_____ Meat   ☐ Prayer

_____ Bread   ☐ Bible Study

_____ Vegetable   ☐ Scripture Reading

_____ Fruit   ☐ Memory Verse

_____ Milk   ☐ Encouragement

_____ Fat   _____ Water

Exercise

Aerobic _____

Strength _____

Flexibility _____

Morning _____

Midday _____

Evening _____

Snacks _____

_____ Meat   ☐ Prayer

_____ Bread   ☐ Bible Study

_____ Vegetable   ☐ Scripture Reading

_____ Fruit   ☐ Memory Verse

_____ Milk   ☐ Encouragement

_____ Fat   _____ Water

Exercise

Aerobic _____

Strength _____

Flexibility _____

DAY 1: Date _____

Morning _____

Midday _____

Evening _____

Snacks _____

____ Meat	☐ Prayer
____ Bread	☐ Bible Study
____ Vegetable	☐ Scripture Reading
____ Fruit	☐ Memory Verse
____ Milk	☐ Encouragement
____ Fat	____ Water

Exercise

Aerobic _____

Strength _____

Flexibility _____

DAY 2: Date _____

Morning _____

Midday _____

Evening _____

Snacks _____

____ Meat	☐ Prayer
____ Bread	☐ Bible Study
____ Vegetable	☐ Scripture Reading
____ Fruit	☐ Memory Verse
____ Milk	☐ Encouragement
____ Fat	____ Water

Exercise

Aerobic _____

Strength _____

Flexibility _____

DAY 3: Date _____

Morning _____

Midday _____

Evening _____

Snacks _____

____ Meat	☐ Prayer
____ Bread	☐ Bible Study
____ Vegetable	☐ Scripture Reading
____ Fruit	☐ Memory Verse
____ Milk	☐ Encouragement
____ Fat	____ Water

Exercise

Aerobic _____

Strength _____

Flexibility _____

DAY 4: Date _____

Morning _____

Midday _____

Evening _____

Snacks _____

____ Meat	☐ Prayer
____ Bread	☐ Bible Study
____ Vegetable	☐ Scripture Reading
____ Fruit	☐ Memory Verse
____ Milk	☐ Encouragement
____ Fat	____ Water

Exercise

Aerobic _____

Strength _____

Flexibility _____

DAY 5: Date _____   DAY 6: Date _____   DAY 7: Date _____

Name _____
Date _____ through _____
Week # _____ Calorie Level _____

Daily Exchange Plan

Level	Meat	Bread	Veggie	Fruit	Milk	Fat
1200	4-5	5-6	3	2-3	2-3	3-4
1400	5-6	6-7	3-4	3-4	2-3	3-4
1500	5-6	7-8	3-4	3-4	2-3	3-4
1600	6-7	8-9	3-4	3-4	2-3	3-4
1800	6-7	10-11	3-4	3-4	2-3	4-5
2000	6-7	11-12	4-5	4-5	2-3	4-5
2200	7-8	12-13	4-5	4-5	2-3	6-7
2400	8-9	13-14	4-5	4-5	2-3	7-8
2600	9-10	14-15	5	5	2-3	7-8
2800	9-10	15-16	5	5	2-3	9

You may always choose the high range of vegetables and fruits. Limit your high range selections to only one of the following: meat, bread, milk or fat.

Weekly Progress

_____ Loss   _____ Gain   _____ Maintain

_____ Attendance   _____ Bible Study
_____ Prayer   _____ Scripture Reading
_____ Memory Verse   _____ CR
_____ Encouragement:
_____ Exercise
Aerobic _____

Strength _____
Flexibility _____

DAY 5, 6, 7 entries (per day):

Morning _____

Midday _____

Evening _____

Snacks _____

_____ Meat   ☐ Prayer
_____ Bread   ☐ Bible Study
_____ Vegetable   ☐ Scripture Reading
_____ Fruit   ☐ Memory Verse
_____ Milk   ☐ Encouragement
_____ Fat   _____ Water

Exercise
Aerobic _____

Strength _____
Flexibility _____

DAY 1: Date _____

Morning _____

Midday _____

Evening _____

Snacks _____

Meat ___	☐ Prayer
Bread ___	☐ Bible Study
Vegetable ___	☐ Scripture Reading
Fruit ___	☐ Memory Verse
Milk ___	☐ Encouragement
Fat ___	Water ___

Exercise
Aerobic _____
Strength _____
Flexibility _____

DAY 2: Date _____

Morning _____

Midday _____

Evening _____

Snacks _____

Meat ___	☐ Prayer
Bread ___	☐ Bible Study
Vegetable ___	☐ Scripture Reading
Fruit ___	☐ Memory Verse
Milk ___	☐ Encouragement
Fat ___	Water ___

Exercise
Aerobic _____
Strength _____
Flexibility _____

DAY 3: Date _____

Morning _____

Midday _____

Evening _____

Snacks _____

Meat ___	☐ Prayer
Bread ___	☐ Bible Study
Vegetable ___	☐ Scripture Reading
Fruit ___	☐ Memory Verse
Milk ___	☐ Encouragement
Fat ___	Water ___

Exercise
Aerobic _____
Strength _____
Flexibility _____

DAY 4: Date _____

Morning _____

Midday _____

Evening _____

Snacks _____

Meat ___	☐ Prayer
Bread ___	☐ Bible Study
Vegetable ___	☐ Scripture Reading
Fruit ___	☐ Memory Verse
Milk ___	☐ Encouragement
Fat ___	Water ___

Exercise
Aerobic _____
Strength _____
Flexibility _____

FIRST PLACE CR

Name _____

Date _____ through _____

Week # _____ Calorie Level _____

Daily Exchange Plan

Level	Meat	Bread	Veggie	Fruit	Milk	Fat
1200	4-5	5-6	3	2-3	2-3	3-4
1400	5-6	6-7	3-4	3-4	2-3	3-4
1500	5-6	7-8	3-4	3-4	2-3	3-4
1600	6-7	8-9	3-4	3-4	2-3	3-4
1800	6-7	10-11	3-4	3-4	2-3	4-5
2000	6-7	11-12	4-5	4-5	2-3	4-5
2200	7-8	12-13	4-5	4-5	2-3	6-7
2400	8-9	13-14	4-5	4-5	2-3	7-8
2600	9-10	14-15	5	5	2-3	7-8
2800	9-10	15-16	5	5	2-3	9

You may always choose the high range of vegetables and fruits. Limit your high range selections to only one of the following: meat, bread, milk or fat.

Weekly Progress

_____ Loss _____ Gain _____ Maintain

_____ Attendance _____ Bible Study
_____ Prayer _____ Scripture Reading
_____ Memory Verse _____ CR
_____ Encouragement:
_____ Exercise
Aerobic

Strength
Flexibility

DAY 5: Date _____

Morning _____

Midday _____

Evening _____

Snacks _____

_____ Meat   ☐ Prayer
_____ Bread   ☐ Bible Study
_____ Vegetable   ☐ Scripture Reading
_____ Fruit   ☐ Memory Verse
_____ Milk   ☐ Encouragement
_____ Fat   ☐ Water
Exercise
Aerobic _____

Strength _____
Flexibility _____

DAY 6: Date _____

Morning _____

Midday _____

Evening _____

Snacks _____

_____ Meat   ☐ Prayer
_____ Bread   ☐ Bible Study
_____ Vegetable   ☐ Scripture Reading
_____ Fruit   ☐ Memory Verse
_____ Milk   ☐ Encouragement
_____ Fat   ☐ Water
Exercise
Aerobic _____

Strength _____
Flexibility _____

DAY 7: Date _____

Morning _____

Midday _____

Evening _____

Snacks _____

_____ Meat   ☐ Prayer
_____ Bread   ☐ Bible Study
_____ Vegetable   ☐ Scripture Reading
_____ Fruit   ☐ Memory Verse
_____ Milk   ☐ Encouragement
_____ Fat   ☐ Water
Exercise
Aerobic _____

Strength _____
Flexibility _____

DAY 1: Date _____

Morning _____

Midday _____

Evening _____

Snacks _____

___ Meat ___	☐ Prayer
___ Bread ___	☐ Bible Study
___ Vegetable ___	☐ Scripture Reading
___ Fruit ___	☐ Memory Verse
___ Milk ___	☐ Encouragement
___ Fat ___ Water ___	

Exercise
Aerobic _____

Strength _____

Flexibility _____

DAY 2: Date _____

Morning _____

Midday _____

Evening _____

Snacks _____

___ Meat ___	☐ Prayer
___ Bread ___	☐ Bible Study
___ Vegetable ___	☐ Scripture Reading
___ Fruit ___	☐ Memory Verse
___ Milk ___	☐ Encouragement
___ Fat ___ Water ___	

Exercise
Aerobic _____

Strength _____

Flexibility _____

DAY 3: Date _____

Morning _____

Midday _____

Evening _____

Snacks _____

___ Meat ___	☐ Prayer
___ Bread ___	☐ Bible Study
___ Vegetable ___	☐ Scripture Reading
___ Fruit ___	☐ Memory Verse
___ Milk ___	☐ Encouragement
___ Fat ___ Water ___	

Exercise
Aerobic _____

Strength _____

Flexibility _____

DAY 4: Date _____

Morning _____

Midday _____

Evening _____

Snacks _____

___ Meat ___	☐ Prayer
___ Bread ___	☐ Bible Study
___ Vegetable ___	☐ Scripture Reading
___ Fruit ___	☐ Memory Verse
___ Milk ___	☐ Encouragement
___ Fat ___ Water ___	

Exercise
Aerobic _____

Strength _____

Flexibility _____

FIRST PLACE CR

DAY 5: Date _____	DAY 6: Date _____	DAY 7: Date _____

Name _____
Date _____ through _____
Week # _____ Calorie Level _____

Daily Exchange Plan

Level	Meat	Bread	Veggie	Fruit	Milk	Fat
1200	4-5	5-6	3	2-3	2-3	3-4
1400	5-6	6-7	3-4	3-4	2-3	3-4
1500	5-6	7-8	3-4	3-4	2-3	3-4
1600	6-7	8-9	3-4	3-4	2-3	3-4
1800	6-7	10-11	3-4	3-4	2-3	3-4
2000	6-7	11-12	4-5	4-5	2-3	4-5
2200	7-8	12-13	4-5	4-5	2-3	6-7
2400	8-9	13-14	4-5	4-5	2-3	7-8
2600	9-10	14-15	5	5	2-3	7-8
2800	9-10	15-16	5	5	2-3	9

You may always choose the high range of vegetables and fruits. Limit your high range selections to only one of the following: meat, bread, milk or fat.

Weekly Progress

____ Loss ____ Gain ____ Maintain

____ Attendance ____ Bible Study
____ Prayer ____ Scripture Reading
____ Memory Verse ____ CR
____ Encouragement:
____ Exercise
Aerobic _____

Strength _____
Flexibility _____

DAY 5: Date _____

Morning _____

Midday _____

Evening _____

Snacks _____

____ Meat _____ ☐ Prayer
____ Bread _____ ☐ Bible Study
____ Vegetable _____ ☐ Scripture Reading
____ Fruit _____ ☐ Memory Verse
____ Milk _____ ☐ Encouragement
____ Fat _____ ☐ Water
Exercise
Aerobic _____

Strength _____
Flexibility _____

DAY 6: Date _____

Morning _____

Midday _____

Evening _____

Snacks _____

____ Meat _____ ☐ Prayer
____ Bread _____ ☐ Bible Study
____ Vegetable _____ ☐ Scripture Reading
____ Fruit _____ ☐ Memory Verse
____ Milk _____ ☐ Encouragement
____ Fat _____ ☐ Water
Exercise
Aerobic _____

Strength _____
Flexibility _____

DAY 7: Date _____

Morning _____

Midday _____

Evening _____

Snacks _____

____ Meat _____ ☐ Prayer
____ Bread _____ ☐ Bible Study
____ Vegetable _____ ☐ Scripture Reading
____ Fruit _____ ☐ Memory Verse
____ Milk _____ ☐ Encouragement
____ Fat _____ ☐ Water
Exercise
Aerobic _____

Strength _____
Flexibility _____

DAY 1: Date _____

Morning _____

Midday _____

Evening _____

Snacks _____

Meat _____ ☐ Prayer
Bread _____ ☐ Bible Study
Vegetable _____ ☐ Scripture Reading
Fruit _____ ☐ Memory Verse
Milk _____ ☐ Encouragement
Fat _____ Water _____

Exercise
Aerobic _____
Strength _____
Flexibility _____

DAY 2: Date _____

Morning _____

Midday _____

Evening _____

Snacks _____

Meat _____ ☐ Prayer
Bread _____ ☐ Bible Study
Vegetable _____ ☐ Scripture Reading
Fruit _____ ☐ Memory Verse
Milk _____ ☐ Encouragement
Fat _____ Water _____

Exercise
Aerobic _____
Strength _____
Flexibility _____

DAY 3: Date _____

Morning _____

Midday _____

Evening _____

Snacks _____

Meat _____ ☐ Prayer
Bread _____ ☐ Bible Study
Vegetable _____ ☐ Scripture Reading
Fruit _____ ☐ Memory Verse
Milk _____ ☐ Encouragement
Fat _____ Water _____

Exercise
Aerobic _____
Strength _____
Flexibility _____

DAY 4: Date _____

Morning _____

Midday _____

Evening _____

Snacks _____

Meat _____ ☐ Prayer
Bread _____ ☐ Bible Study
Vegetable _____ ☐ Scripture Reading
Fruit _____ ☐ Memory Verse
Milk _____ ☐ Encouragement
Fat _____ Water _____

Exercise
Aerobic _____
Strength _____
Flexibility _____

FIRST PLACE CR

Name _____

Date _____ through _____

Week # _____ Calorie Level _____

Daily Exchange Plan

Level	Meat	Bread	Veggie	Fruit	Milk	Fat
1200	4-5	5-6	3	2-3	2-3	3-4
1400	5-6	6-7	3-4	3-4	2-3	3-4
1500	5-6	7-8	3-4	3-4	2-3	3-4
1600	6-7	8-9	3-4	3-4	2-3	3-4
1800	6-7	10-11	3-4	3-4	2-3	4-5
2000	6-7	11-12	4-5	4-5	2-3	4-5
2200	7-8	12-13	4-5	4-5	2-3	6-7
2400	8-9	13-14	4-5	4-5	2-3	7-8
2600	9-10	14-15	5	5	2-3	7-8
2800	9-10	15-16	5	5	2-3	9

You may always choose the high range of vegetables and fruits. Limit your high range selections to only one of the following: meat, bread, milk or fat.

Weekly Progress

____ Loss ____ Gain ____ Maintain

____ Attendance   ____ Bible Study
____ Prayer   ____ Scripture Reading
____ Memory Verse ____ CR
____ Encouragement:
____ Exercise
Aerobic _____

Strength _____
Flexibility _____

DAY 5: Date _____

Morning _____

Midday _____

Evening _____

Snacks _____

____ Meat   ☐ Prayer
____ Bread   ☐ Bible Study
____ Vegetable   ☐ Scripture Reading
____ Fruit   ☐ Memory Verse
____ Milk   ☐ Encouragement
____ Fat   ☐ Water

Exercise
Aerobic _____

Strength _____
Flexibility _____

DAY 6: Date _____

Morning _____

Midday _____

Evening _____

Snacks _____

____ Meat   ☐ Prayer
____ Bread   ☐ Bible Study
____ Vegetable   ☐ Scripture Reading
____ Fruit   ☐ Memory Verse
____ Milk   ☐ Encouragement
____ Fat   ☐ Water

Exercise
Aerobic _____

Strength _____
Flexibility _____

DAY 7: Date _____

Morning _____

Midday _____

Evening _____

Snacks _____

____ Meat   ☐ Prayer
____ Bread   ☐ Bible Study
____ Vegetable   ☐ Scripture Reading
____ Fruit   ☐ Memory Verse
____ Milk   ☐ Encouragement
____ Fat   ☐ Water

Exercise
Aerobic _____

Strength _____
Flexibility _____

DAY 1: Date _____

Morning _____

Midday _____

Evening _____

Snacks _____

- Meat _____
- Bread _____
- Vegetable _____
- Fruit _____
- Milk _____
- Fat _____ Water _____

☐ Prayer
☐ Bible Study
☐ Scripture Reading
☐ Memory Verse
☐ Encouragement

Exercise
Aerobic _____
Strength _____
Flexibility _____

DAY 2: Date _____

Morning _____

Midday _____

Evening _____

Snacks _____

- Meat _____
- Bread _____
- Vegetable _____
- Fruit _____
- Milk _____
- Fat _____ Water _____

☐ Prayer
☐ Bible Study
☐ Scripture Reading
☐ Memory Verse
☐ Encouragement

Exercise
Aerobic _____
Strength _____
Flexibility _____

DAY 3: Date _____

Morning _____

Midday _____

Evening _____

Snacks _____

- Meat _____
- Bread _____
- Vegetable _____
- Fruit _____
- Milk _____
- Fat _____ Water _____

☐ Prayer
☐ Bible Study
☐ Scripture Reading
☐ Memory Verse
☐ Encouragement

Exercise
Aerobic _____
Strength _____
Flexibility _____

DAY 4: Date _____

Morning _____

Midday _____

Evening _____

Snacks _____

- Meat _____
- Bread _____
- Vegetable _____
- Fruit _____
- Milk _____
- Fat _____ Water _____

☐ Prayer
☐ Bible Study
☐ Scripture Reading
☐ Memory Verse
☐ Encouragement

Exercise
Aerobic _____
Strength _____
Flexibility _____

CONTRIBUTORS

Kay Smith, the writer of the Wellness Worksheet for this study, is the associate national director of First Place. Having served on staff at First Baptist Church—the birthplace of the First Place program—in Houston, Texas, since 1987, Kay is also a popular speaker at retreats, seminars, conferences, fitness weeks and workshops across the country. Her delightful personality and love for people endear her to everyone she meets. Kay and her husband, Joe, live in Roscoe, Texas, and have two children and five grandchildren.

Scott Wilson, C.E.C., A.A.C., the author of the menu plans for this study, has been cooking professionally for 23 years. A certified executive chef with the American Culinary Federation, he currently works in the Greater Atlanta area as a personal chef and food consultant and is a certified personal chef with the United States Personal Chef Association. Along with serving as the national food consultant for First Place, he is on the culinary program advisory board of the Art Institute in Atlanta. Scott has also authored two cookbooks, *Dining Under the Magnolia* and *Healthy Home Cooking*. He is also active in church work and enjoys spending time with his wife of 18 years, Jennifer, and their daughter, Katie.

THE BIBLE'S WAY TO WEIGHT LOSS

The Bible-Based Weight-Loss Program
Used Successfully by Over a Half Million People!

Are you one of the millions of disheartened dieters who've tried one fad diet after another without success? If so, your search for a successful diet is over! First Place is the proven weight-loss program, born over 20 years ago in the First Baptist Church of Houston.

But First Place does much more than help you take off weight and keep it off. This Bible-based program will transform your life in every way—physically, mentally, spiritually and emotionally. Now's the time to join!

ESSENTIAL FIRST PLACE PROGRAM MATERIALS

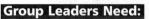

Group Leaders Need:

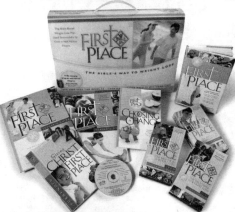

■ **Group Starter Kit** • *ISBN 08307.28708*

This kit has everything group leaders need to help others change their lives forever by giving Christ first place!

Kit includes:

- *Leader's Guide*
- *Member's Guide*
- *Giving Christ First Place Bible Study* with Scripture Memory Music CD
- *Choosing to Change* by Carole Lewis
- *First Place* by Carole Lewis with Terry Whalin
- *Orientation* Video
- *Nine Commitments* Video
- *Food Exchange Plan* Video
- *An Introduction to First Place* Video

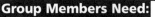

Group Members Need:

■ **Member's Kit** • *ISBN 08307.28694*

All the material is easy to understand and spells out principles members can easily apply in their daily lives.

Kit includes:

- *Member's Guide* • *Choosing to Change* by Carole Lewis
- 13 Commitment Records • Four Motivational Audiocassettes
- *Prayer Journal*
- *Walking in the Word:* Scripture Memory Verses

■ **First Place Bible Study**

Giving Christ First Place Bible Study with Scripture Memory Music CD

Bible Study ISBN 08307.28643

Many other First Place Bible studies are available. Visit www.firstplace.org for a complete listing

Available where Christian books are sold or by calling **1-800-4-GOSPEL**.
Join the First Place community at www.firstplace.org

Gospel Light

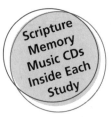
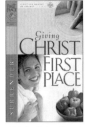
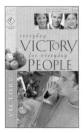
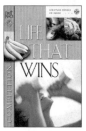
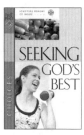
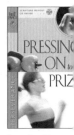
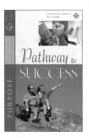
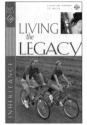
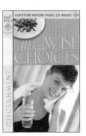
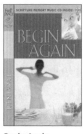
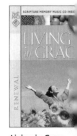

Inspiration
& Information
Everymonth
Subscribe Today!

Every newsletter gives you:
- ### New recipes
- ### Helpful articles
- ### Food tips
- ### Inspiring testimonies
- ### Coming events
- ### And much more!

**Register for our FREE
e-newsletter at
www.firstplace.org**

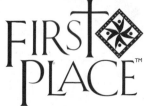

Must-Have Publication for all First Place Leaders & Members!

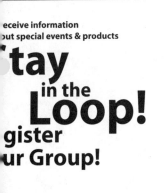